A Colour Atlas of

DISEASES & DISORDERS OF THE DOMESTIC FOWL & TURKEY

Second Edition

C. J. Randall

MA VetMB MRCVS
Ministry of Agriculture, Fisheries and Food
Lasswade Veterinary Laboratory
Edinburgh, Scotland

Wolfe Publishing Ltd

© Crown copyright 1991
© illustrations **167–170** Dr R C Jones
Second edition published by Wolfe Publishing Ltd 1991
Printed by BPCC Hazell Books, Aylesbury, England
ISBN 0 7234 1628 1
First edition published by Wolfe Medical Publications Ltd 1985

A CIP catalogue record for this book is available from the British Library.

This book is one of the titles in the series of Wolfe Atlases, a series that
brings together the world's largest systematic published collection of
diagnostic colour photographs.

For a full list of Atlases in the series, plus forthcoming titles and details of
our surgical, dental and veterinary Atlases, please write to Wolfe
Publishing Ltd, 2–16 Torrington Place, London WC1E 7LT, England.

CONTENTS

PREFACE

The original idea of the Atlas – to provide the diagnostician with photographs of the main post-mortem and histopathological features of common diseases in the domestic fowl and turkey – remains unchanged. The Atlas does not aim to cover the other procedures that may be required to confirm a diagnosis. Although some of the original photographs have been replaced and some sections have been expanded as better examples of lesions have arisen, the format nevertheless follows that of the first edition. The text has been altered where necessary and the opportunity has been taken to make minor changes and corrections. Photographs of moult, feather wear and vibrionic hepatitis have been omitted. Several disorders that either were not selected for the first edition or have since emerged as being of importance are now included. The diseases described in the Atlas continue to reflect the author's experience. Amongst the new illustrations there are occasional further examples of lesions in avian species other than the fowl and turkey.

Difficulties remain in the selection of suitable names for poorly defined diseases or for those where particular clinical signs or post-mortem appearances have been adopted as syndromes in the literature. Names such as 'sudden death syndrome' and 'swollen head syndrome' have been retained because they are in general use, but it is acknowledged that this usage is not ideal.

As in the first edition, diseases that might usefully be considered together are arranged under main group headings rather than being listed alphabetically. Again, there is a miscellaneous group of conditions whose aetiologies are generally understood, as well as a large section on diseases of uncertain or unknown cause. Included in the latter are right ventricular heart failure in broilers and the infectious stunting syndrome. Although knowledge of the pathogenesis of both has increased since publication of the first edition, there are still uncertainties about the causes in different countries, and they have therefore been left in this category.

It is hoped that the diagnostician may find it more useful to see photographs of a particular disease grouped together rather than placed in a systematic arrangement under bodily systems, so that, for example, not all the illustrations of kidney abnormalities are confined to the section on renal failure. Elsewhere, more attention has been given to bacterial osteomyelitis, reflecting its importance, but following the general arrangement it is illustrated under different headings. There are other similar anomalies but the intention throughout has been to make it easier to consider aspects of differential diagnosis.

All photomicrographs are of tissue sections stained with haematoxylin and eosin, unless stated otherwise. Where, occasionally, water-soluble acrylic resins have been used for tissue embedding to show particular features, this is indicated in the accompanying legends.

ACKNOWLEDGEMENTS

I remain indebted to all those friends and colleagues acknowledged previously who helped with, or contributed to, the first edition.

I am most grateful to Dr S R I Duff, Agricultural Food and Research Council, Institute for Grassland and Animal Production, Dr M Pattison, the Hellig, Pattison and Jones Partnership, Dr R L Reece, Agricultural Food and Research Council, Houghton Laboratory, and Dr C Riddell, Western College of Veterinary Medicine, University of Saskatchewan, for reading the draft manuscript, for discussions on different aspects of disease, and for their many helpful comments. I also thank Dr Duff for contributing the two illustrations at **293** and Dr Riddell for giving the tissue section from which the photograph **332** was prepared. Dr R J Julian, University of Guelph, is thanked for several discussions about poultry disease and for suggesting 'cholangiohepatitis' as a name for the disease in broilers illustrated in **338–342**. A number of helpful amendments to the legends of photographs in the first edition were suggested by Dr F T W Jordan, University of Liverpool, to whom I also express my thanks.

Transparencies that were kindly provided for the first edition have again been used: I thank the late Dr J E Wilson, previously Director of the Veterinary Laboratory, Lasswade, for **86**, **87**, **89–91**, **130**, **187**, **200**, **239**, and **331**; Dr R C Jones, Department of Veterinary Pathology, University of Liverpool, for **167–170** (copyright of these four pictures rests with Dr R C Jones); and Mr D E Gray, lately Librarian at the Central Veterinary Laboratory, for arranging the loan of **67**, **92–94**, **108**, **135**, **137**, **140** and **141** from the Library's collection. Sections of reticuloendotheliosis virus induced tumours in turkeys (**211**) and erythroid leukosis (**201**) were generously given, respectively, by Dr J S McDougall, Houghton Poultry Research Station, and by the late Dr J G Campbell.

The journal, *Avian Pathology*, is thanked for permission to publish **232**. I also thank Mr R K Field for photographing the specimen in **333**.

I am indebted to the staff of the Lasswade Veterinary Laboratory. In particular, I thank the members of the Pathology Section for producing excellent slides for the purposes of photomicrography, and also Mrs I I G Stenhouse and Mrs M D Forbes for typing the manuscript and patiently accommodating the many changes.

BACTERIAL DISEASES

Coli bacillosis
(including peritonitis in layers and salpingitis)

1 Coli septicaemia. Polyserositis caused by *Escherichia coli*. Severe pericarditis, perihepatitis and air sacculitis in a broiler following primary viral infection of the respiratory tract. The fibrinous exudate covering one lobe of the liver has been cut to show the surface of the organ beneath. Hepatic and particularly pericardial lesions of this type may be seen in some systemic salmonella infections in young chickens and turkeys (*see* **85**).

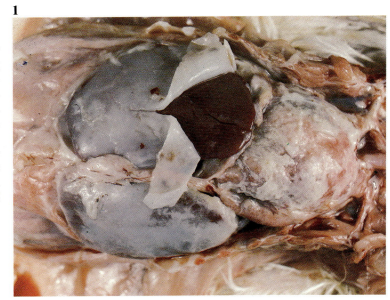

2 Coli septicaemia. Liver section showing the fibrinous nature of the deposit (arrow) on the surface of the organ. This lesion arises from inflammation of the hepatic peritoneal sac. Martius scarlet blue.

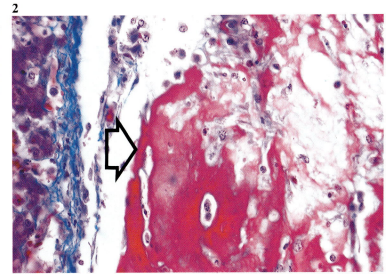

3 Coli septicaemia. Multiple splenic periarteriolar lesions contain prominent eosinophilic coagulum in H & E (haematoxylin and eosin) stained sections but in these prints Martius scarlet blue is used to demonstrate the fibrinous nature of the exudate. This feature is frequently encountered in cases of Coli septicaemia. It is usually marked in this infection but similar changes may occur in other septicaemias and viraemias. Low- and high-power fields are shown.

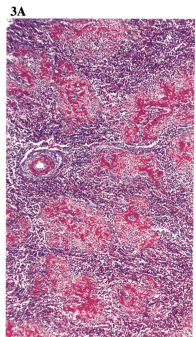

3A

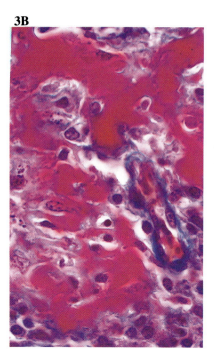

3B

4 Coli septicaemia. Fibrinous thrombi (arrows) in hepatic sinusoids of a young turkey (*see also* **375A**). Again, a common feature of this disease but also seen in other septicaemias.

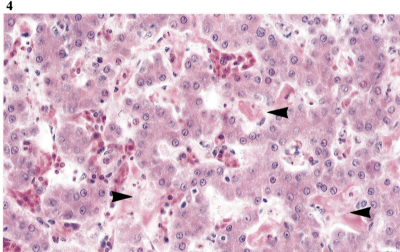

4

5 Coli septicaemia. A higher-power view of **4**. The thrombi have been stained with phosphotungstic acid haematoxylin, imparting a blue-black colour to the fibrinous component.

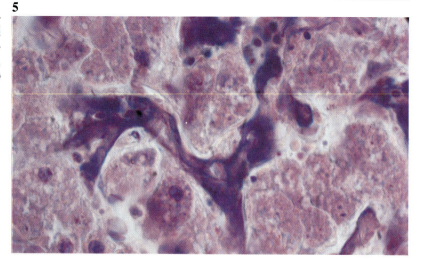

5

6 Coli septicaemia. Synovitis of hock joints is commonly found in broilers. The articular exudate is usually thick and cream-coloured. It may also, as here, be tinged a reddish-brown. Concurrent lesions of osteomyelitis may be present, particularly at the proximal tibiotarsal growth plate (*see* **29**, **43**).

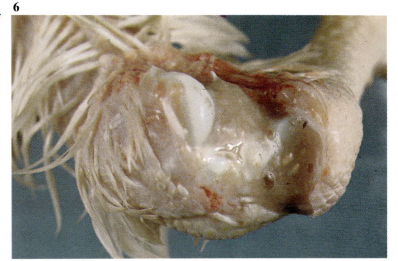

7 Coli septicaemia. Salpingitis in a 3-week-old broiler. Inflammation of the immature oviduct is a relatively common finding in broilers.

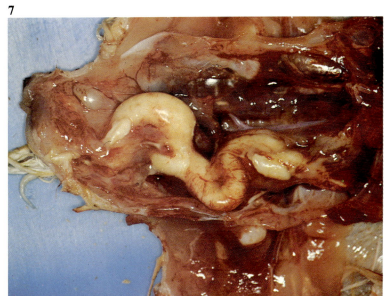

8 Coli septicaemia. Turkey grower. Lesions were confined in this instance to an overall carcase congestion and a marked congestion of the spleen (arrow). This bird gave a serologically positive reaction for *Mycoplasma meleagridis* antibodies. In this species pericarditis may accompany Coli septicaemia, but fibrinous deposits on the liver are less common. Greening of the liver may occur after exposure to the air.

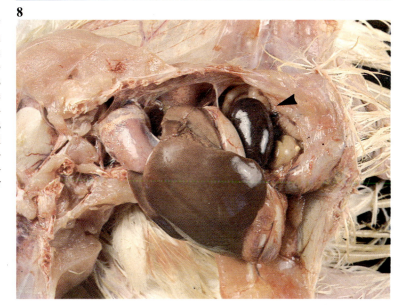

9 *E. coli* is isolated from the great majority of cases of peritonitis in adult laying fowl, as either a primary or a secondary invader. The lesion is often called 'egg peritonitis', but the presence of yolk mixed with the exudate is variable. Birds dying in acute stages are usually septicaemic.

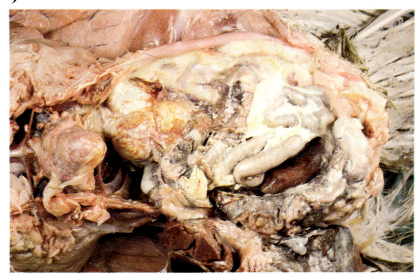

10 Laying fowl may die as a result of acute peritonitis. Many survive this episode, with the result that the inflammatory exudate becomes partly organised. The affected oviducts may be extremely enlarged and occupy most of the abdominal cavity. *E. coli* is most frequently isolated from such lesions. Organisms such as *Staphylococcus aureus* and *Pasteurella haemolytica* are amongst other bacteria that may be isolated in either pure or mixed culture, particularly from acute cases.

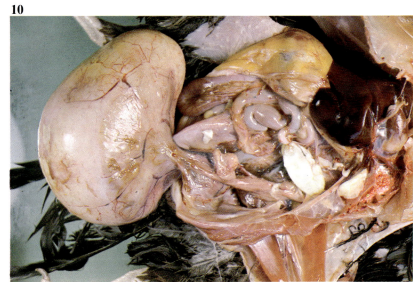

11 The exudate contained within the oviduct of **10** has been cut to show the onion-layered texture of the inflammatory exudate and, in this case, a shelled egg.

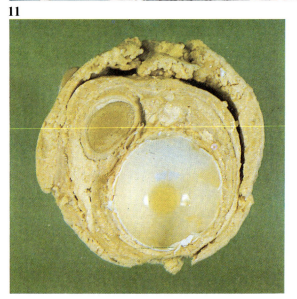

12 Layering of the exudate within an oviduct. Small basophilically staining clumps of bacteria are visible. Their presence is variable.

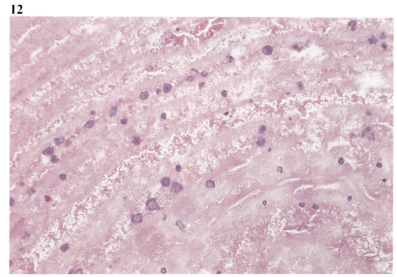

13 A band of blue-black fibrinous material within oviduct exudate. Phosphotungstic acid haematoxylin.

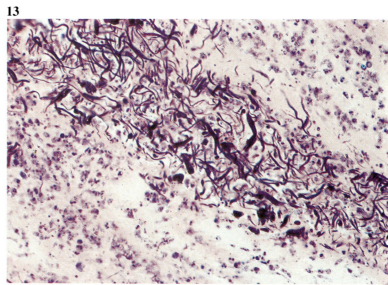

14 Coli granuloma (Hjärres disease) affecting the caeca of a laying fowl. The lesions must be distinguished from those of tuberculosis, which is best done histologically (*see* **73**).

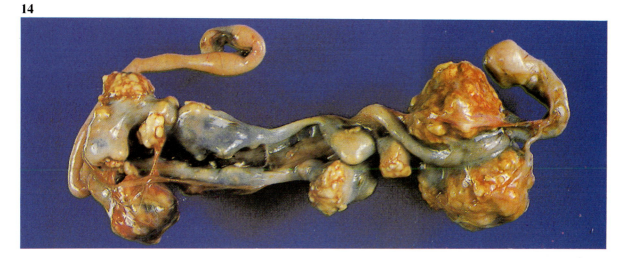

15 Coli granuloma. Cross-section of a granuloma from **14**.

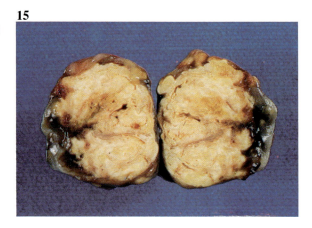

Fowl cholera (*Pasteurella multocida*)

16 Swollen wattles in a male broiler breeder due to *P. multocida* infection. The affected males may be slightly depressed in localised infection of this type. Swollen wattles may also occur amongst the females, as well as a cellulitis, which is usually seen over the head and neck. Otitis, with the appearance of exudate at the external ear opening, is less common.

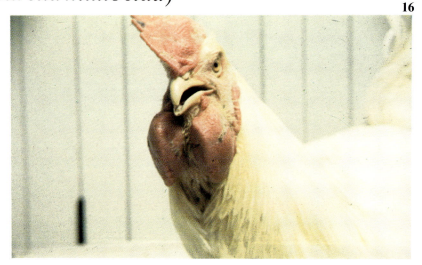

17 Core of purulent material in a swollen wattle of a broiler breeder hen. *P. multocida* can be isolated from most acute lesions of this type but only rarely from chronic abscesses. This may give rise to some diagnostic difficulty as wattle abscesses can be caused by a variety of bacteria.

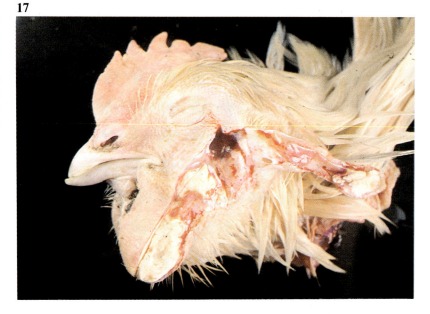

18

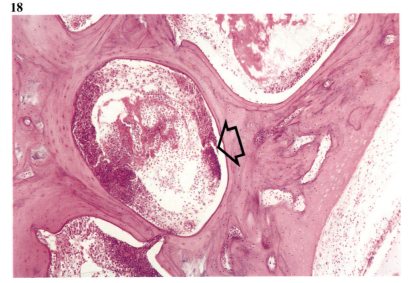

18 Severe inflammation of the air spaces within the spongy bone of the skull may be encountered in some cranial forms of *P. multocida* infection. Here, purulent exudate is present within such an air space (arrow). Grossly, this form of the disease may resemble the swollen head syndrome in broiler fowl and should be distinguished from it (*see* **416**).

19

19 Purulent synovitis in a hock joint of an adult broiler breeder cockerel. Lameness may be a presenting clinical sign in some outbreaks.

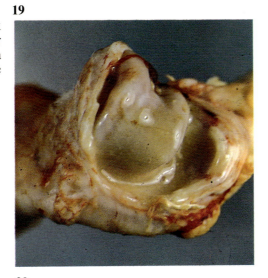

20

20 Comparison of, on the right, pale-flecked exudate from a case of acute staphylococcal synovitis with, on the left, the more yellow-tinged granular exudate obtained from a *P. multocida*-infected joint.

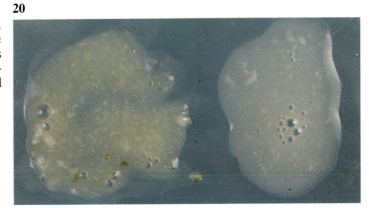

21 Peritonitis is often found in adult layers in septicaemic forms of the infection.

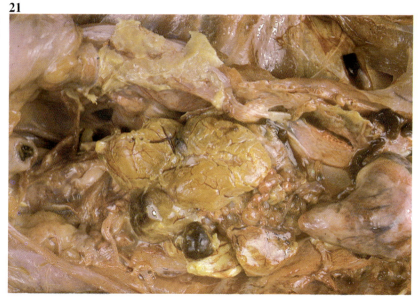

22 Blood-stained mucus in the mouth of a septicaemic turkey breeder.

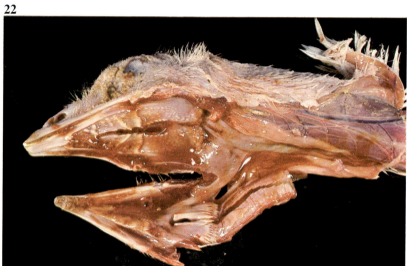

23 Purulent pleuropneumonia in a 10-week-old turkey. This bird was unvaccinated. Pneumonic lesions are more commonly seen in turkeys but, if they do occur in the fowl, pulmonary oedema may be a prominent feature.

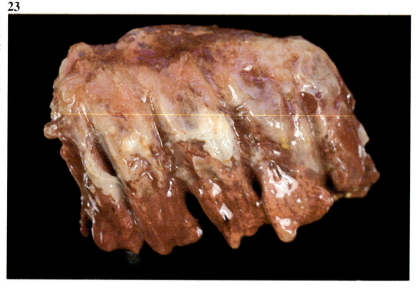

24 Cross-section from the lung illustrated in **23**, showing consolidated areas of pneumonia.

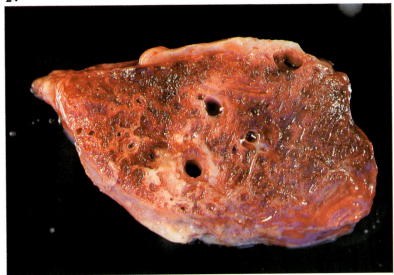

25 Acutely inflamed, necrotic parabronchus in the lung of a 12-week-old turkey. Fibrinopurulent exudate is present in the airway. Note the incomplete ring of basophilically staining bacteria near the periphery of the lesion.

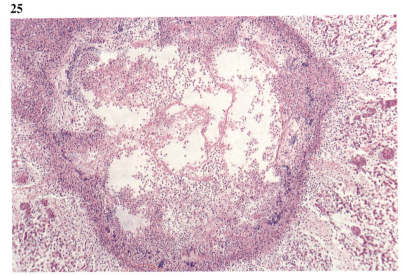

26 Masses of pasteurella organisms within a lung of a turkey that died from a dual infection of *P. multocida* and Newcastle disease.

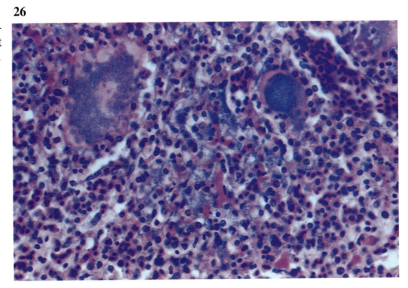

27 Acute pneumonia in a 22-week-old broiler breeder. Pasteurella organisms usually stain more basophilically (arrow) in H & E preparations than most other commonly encountered Gram-negative bacteria. The tissue to the right of the bacteria is necrotic, that to the left reactive.

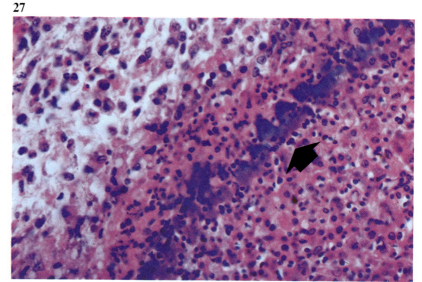

Pseudotuberculosis (*Yersinia pseudotuberculosis*)

28 Large purulent osteomyelitic focus in the proximal femur of a 12-week-old turkey. Lameness was the main clinical sign in a severe outbreak on the farm of origin. Knee joints contained pale yellow viscous exudate. Focal hepatic and splenic lesions were seen less frequently than bone marrow and joint abnormalities in this incident. The disease is uncommon.

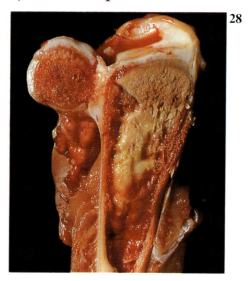

29 Lesions of acute osteomyelitis were seen in another outbreak in the form of small gelatinous metaphyseal foci. This appearance may be observed in other bacterial infections. Proximal tibiotarsus, 14-week-old turkey.

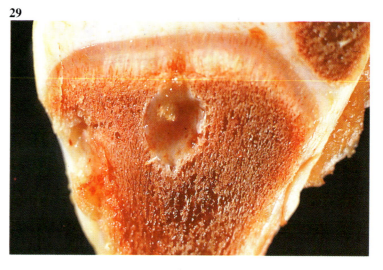

30 Liver discoloration and mottling in a 12-week-old turkey. This appearance may be encountered at meat inspection, usually in carcases that have bled imperfectly. Bacterial osteomyelitis should be considered in the differential diagnosis and a careful search made for lesions by splitting the long bones in several planes. Several types of infection, such as staphylococci, *Escherichia coli* and *Y. pseudotuberculosis* (as here), may be involved.

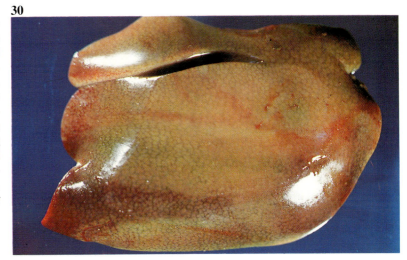

31 A liver such as that illustrated in **30** is usually affected by a diffuse hepatitis. Large numbers of leucocytes, particularly granulocytes, are often visible in the hepatic sinusoids (lower **31A**). Another feature seen here is the presence of ceroid within Kupffer cell cytoplasm (arrows). This pigment has reacted positively (**31B**) to a long Ziehl-Neelsen stain. Coliform infection, turkey grower.

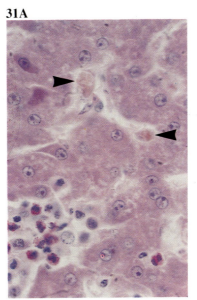

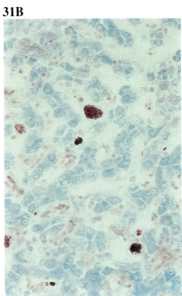

Yolk sac infection and omphalitis

32 The abdomen of this chick is greatly distended as a result of yolk sac infection. Most birds die at 3–4 days of age. The carcases frequently smell unpleasantly.

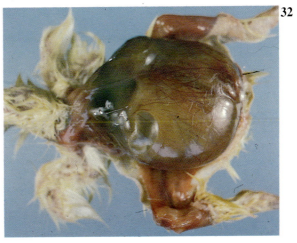

33 Omphalitis often accompanies the infection. Note the marked reddening of the navel tissues in this chick.

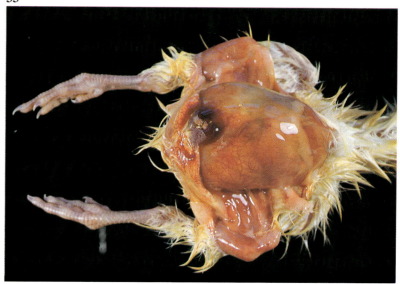

34 Intense inflammation of an infected yolk sac.

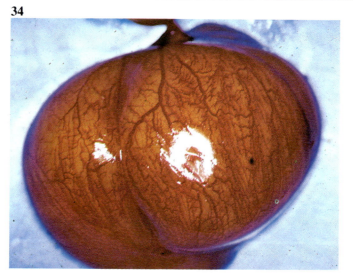

35 The normal consistency of the yolk is lost, and in the acute stages of the disease the contents are thin and have a strong odour. The presence of soft and friable viscera together with moist abdominal skin and down led to the condition being called 'mushy chick disease'.

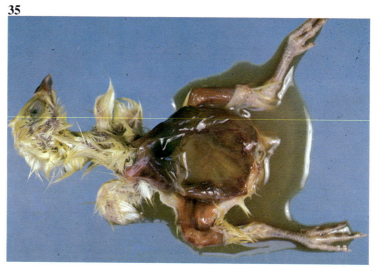

36 Acute inflammation of a yolk sac membrane on the left. Purulent material and poorly staining bacterial clumps (arrows) are to the right.

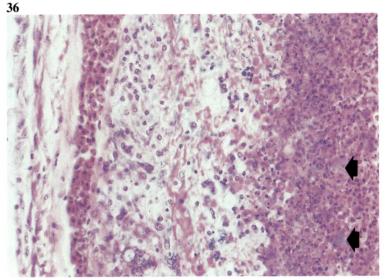

37 The contents of the infected yolk sac may become inspissated if the chick or poult survives into the second week of life. Such sacs are often adherent to the posterior abdominal wall (where they may be palpated in the live bird) or to the viscera. Infected yolk sac remnants containing deeply pigmented caseous material are a frequent incidental post-mortem finding in older birds.

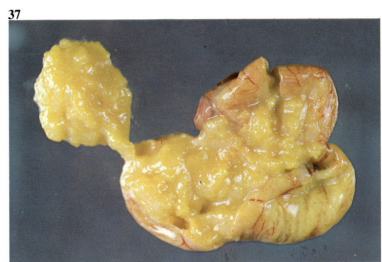

38 Intense lung congestion (arrow) may occur in the acute stages. Note the pool of yolky material within the abdominal cavity. Many chicks dying at this stage have full digestive tracts.

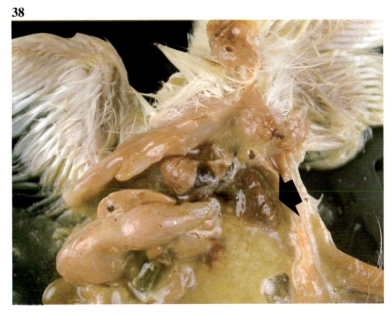

39 A wide variety of bacteria may be isolated in either single or mixed infections. *Escherichia coli* is frequently isolated from affected birds and may lead to classical lesions (*see* **1**) towards the end of the first week. The spleens of such birds are often swollen and congested, and may have abnormal contours due to compression against the surrounding organs. Synovitis and osteomyelitis may also be caused by coliform infections and other organisms introduced by this route.

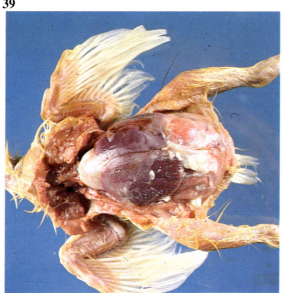

Staphylococcal infection (*Staphylococcus aureus*)

40 Synovitis associated with staphylococcal infection in a 10-week-old broiler breeder. This infection is most often seen during the rearing period. The base of the gastrocnemius tendon is usually swollen as well as the joint. Reoviruses may need to be considered as primary infecting agents in some outbreaks (*see* **167–170**).

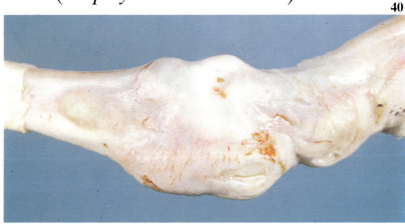

41 The hock joint in **40** has been opened to reveal the large quantity of purulent exudate. Lesions often extend into the sheaths of the digital flexor tendons and the gastrocnemius tendon.

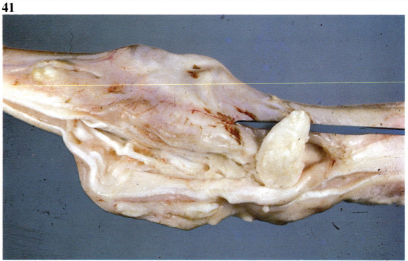

42 Chronic case of staphylococcal arthritis in a young broiler breeder, showing erosion of the cartilage over the distal tibiotarsal condyles.

43 Osteomyelitis in a turkey grower. The infected tissue is pale and crumbly and situated distal (arrows) to the proximal tibiotarsal physis. Osteomyelitis is frequently found at this site in broilers and young turkeys. Staphylococci (and *Escherichia coli*) are often isolated from such lesions. The long bones – particularly the tibiotarsus – should always be split when young birds are presented with a history of lameness. If osteomyelitis is suspected it may be necessary to split bones in several planes in order to identify the lesions. Early stages of infection may be recognised as small grey gelatinous foci (*see* **29**).

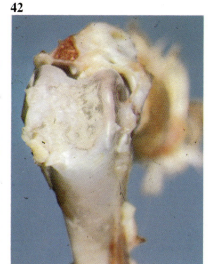

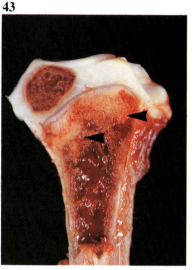

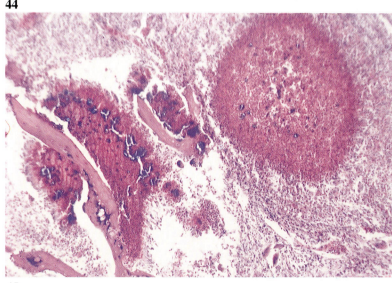

44 Osteomyelitis. A small inflammatory focus containing numerous clusters of bacteria in a proximal tibiotarsal physis of a 6-week-old broiler.

45 Clearly defined necrotic lesions in the liver of a 15-week-old turkey breeder that had been beak-trimmed 10 days previously. There were concurrent lesions of synovitis. Hepatic (and splenic) lesions of this type are commonly seen in laying fowl in association with vegetative endocarditis (*see* **50**). Staphylococcal septicaemias occur from time to time in commercial and breeding hens with few gross lesions other than generalised carcase and hepatic congestion and renal pallor.

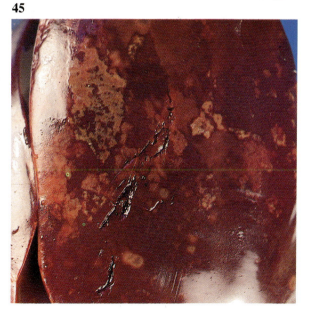

46 Liver lesions similar to those in **45** often contain colonies of strongly basophilic bacteria surrounded by large zones of necrosis.

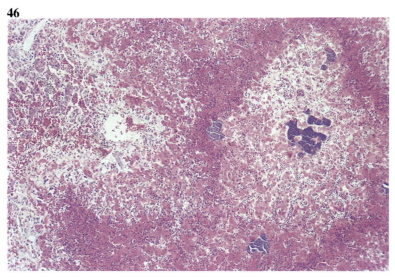

47 Strongly Gram-positive clumps of cocci seen in a lower-power view of **46**. The staining of these bacteria in tissue is sometimes sufficiently intense to give the initial impression of artefacts superimposed on the section.

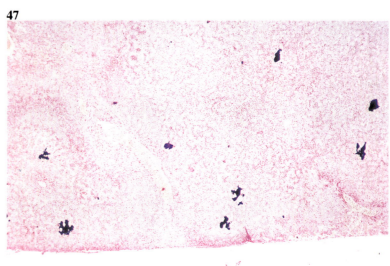

48 Increased numbers of relatively immature granulocytes in periportal tissue of a liver from a broiler breeder with chronically infected hock joints. This feature may indicate the presence of extrahepatic foci of infection, but it is not specific. Acrylic resin.

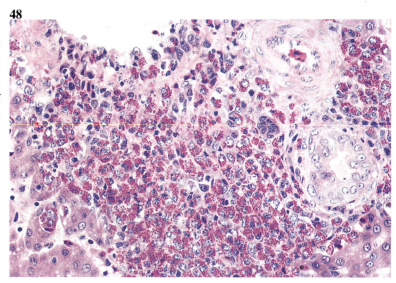

49 Septic embolus in a thrombosed myocardial vessel of an adult commercial layer. Note the basophilic bacteria.

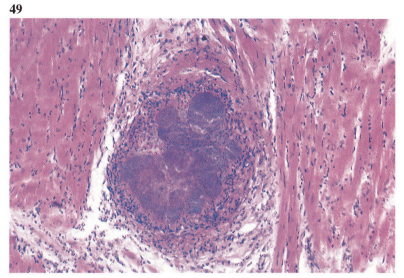

50 Sporadic deaths, particularly in commercial layers, are often caused by vegetative endocarditis. Such lesions are commonest on the left atrioventricular and aortic valves. *Streptococcus* and *Pasteurella* species may also be isolated from vegetative lesions of this type.

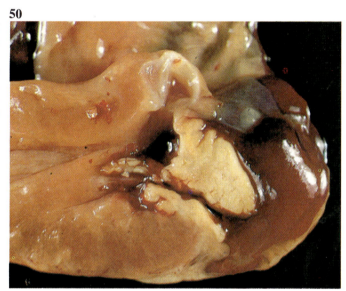

51 Pale swollen anterior division of a kidney in a 7-week-old septicaemic broiler. Lobular outlines are prominent. These features are common non-specific findings in several septicaemias and toxaemias (*see* **59**), and may give rise to a false impression that primary renal disease is present.

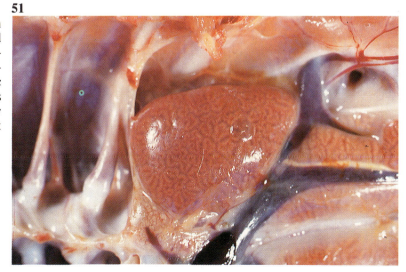

52 Dilation of distal convoluted tubules (arrows) and other distal parts of nephrons, with some flattening of lining epithelium, in a section from the kidney in **51**. The changes are interpreted as a terminal dysfunction with, possibly, urates collecting in the distal tubules (*see* **Renal failure** page 139). Such urates are likely to dissolve during the normal fixation of the tissue. Acrylic resin.

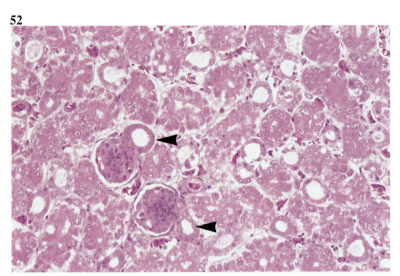

Necrotic enteritis

53 Early necrotic enteritis in the small intestine of a 3-week-old broiler. The mucosal surface is abnormally pale due to necrosis of the tips of the villi.

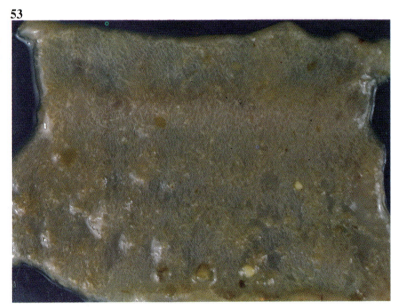

54 Mottling of the serosal surface of the small intestine. The lesion is more advanced than in **53** and is caused by early fissuring of the mucosa. Small flecks of detached mucosa are usually apparent in the intestinal contents by this stage.

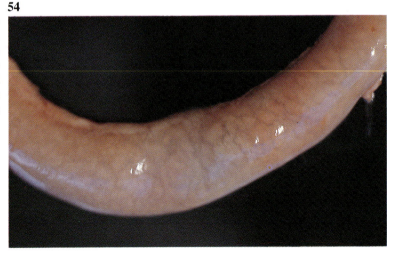

55 Advanced lesion. The necrotic mucous membrane is fissured and detaching from the deeper layers. Most of the upper small intestine is usually involved in the lesion. The disease is seen mainly in young broilers and broiler breeders.

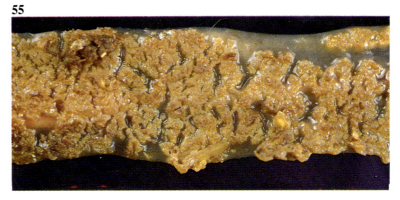

56 Smear of small intestinal contents showing the predominance of Gram-positive bacilli. These organisms are often decaying and stain variably. Profuse growths of *Clostridium perfringens* are isolated from the intestines of birds that have died. Gram.

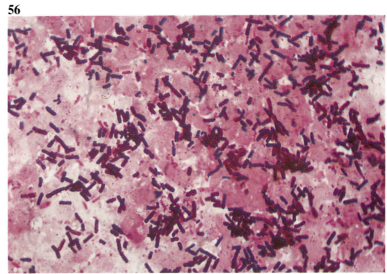

57 Necrosis of the inner part (arrows) of the small intestinal mucosa.

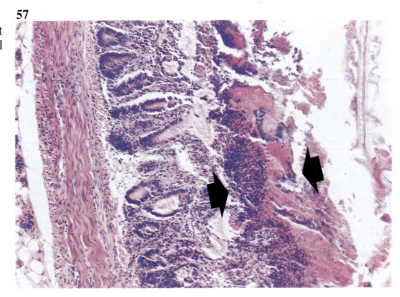

58 This section has been stained by the Gram-Weigert method. Numerous Gram-positive organisms are visible on the surface of the necrotic mucosa on the right. The pink line (arrows) represents the junction of the inner necrotic tissue from the still viable deeper mucosa.

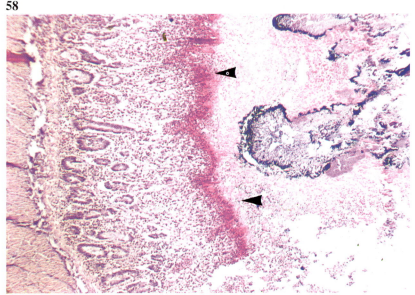

59 Kidneys of birds that have died as a result of necrotic enteritis are usually pale, slightly swollen, and have prominent lobular outlines. Both the gross appearance and histopathological findings are similar to those described under staphylococcal infection (*see* **51**). Although not specific, these are nevertheless useful post-mortem features which may direct attention to other parts of the carcase.

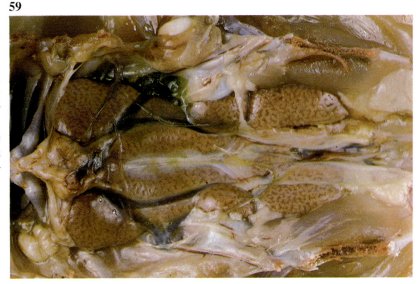

60 Intense congestion of a broiler liver, typical of acute cases. In some instances the clostridia invade the portal blood system *post mortem*, with the result that autolysis is more advanced in the tissue surrounding the intrahepatic veins, which causes focal pallor. Focal hepatic abscessation may occur due to invasion of *C. perfringens* during life, and may be seen at slaughter of broiler flocks that have recovered from the intestinal disease.

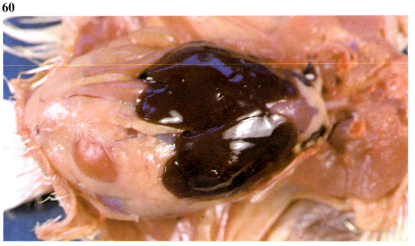

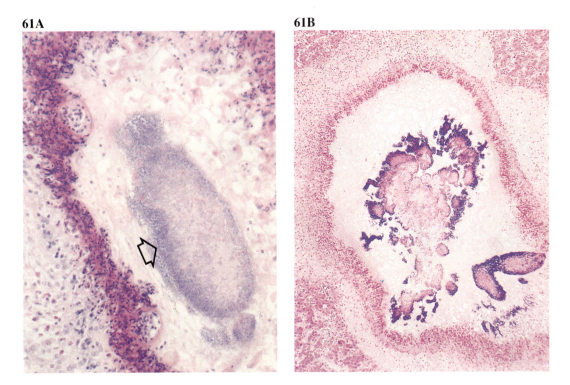

61 Hepatic abscesses in two broilers resulting from *C. perfringens* infection. Note that the periphery of the bacterial clump (arrow, **61A**) is stained more basophilically than at its centre. In a Gram-stained section (**61B**) this corresponds to retention of Gram-positive staining at the rim of the clump but loss of this property centrally.

Gangrenous dermatitis

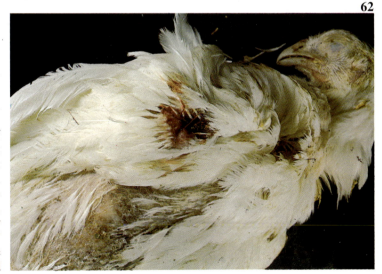

62 A small area of wet inflamed skin is present on this broiler's wing. Lesions like this are variable in size and may be found anywhere on the body. The disease is usually associated with either single or mixed infections of coagulase positive staphylococci and clostridia (e.g. *Clostridium septicum* and *C. perfringens*). During the early part of an outbreak birds may die without obvious lesions affecting the skin, but in some instances small moist sores can be found between the toes. Birds are rarely seen ill. If clostridia are involved, the rate of decomposition may be very rapid – with the result that 'green' carcases can be submitted with the history that the birds have been picked up as freshly dead an hour or two beforehand.

63 When handled *post mortem*, the skin lesions defeather very easily and are usually underrun with gelatinous and sanguinous fluid.

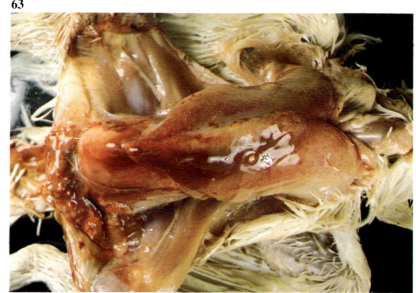

64 Part or all of the lung may undergo liquefaction, particularly when the infection is predominantly staphylococcal. It may be the most notable post-mortem feature of carcases examined at the beginning of outbreaks. Note (in **64A**) the small unaffected areas of tissue at either end. A Gram-stained smear (**64B**) from a similarly affected lung exhibits large numbers of Gram-positive cocci.

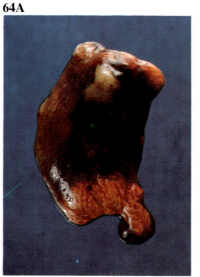

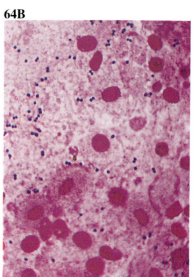

65 Clumps of staphylococci in the necrotic zone of a lung.

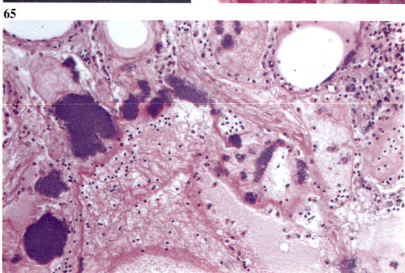

Listeriosis (*Listeria monocytogenes*)

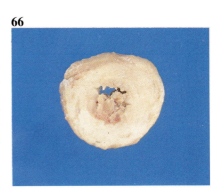

66 Myocarditis in a 7-week-old commercial layer pullet. The heart has been cut through to reveal the almost complete replacement of the myocardium with pale inflammatory tissue. Focal lesions may occur. The disease is uncommon and should not be confused with the lymphoproliferative lesions of Marek's disease that often affect the heart – particularly when necrosis has occurred in the lymphoid tumour, giving rise to yellowish foci within the neoplasm.

Erysipelas (*Erysipelothrix rhusiopathiae*)

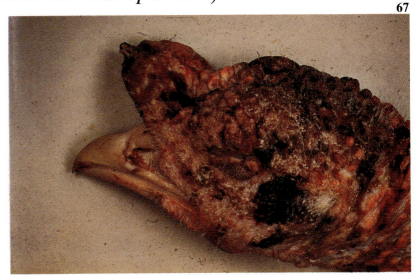

67 The disease is common in turkeys but rare in the fowl. Carcases are congested and show general septicaemic changes. The head of this bird is scabbed. Gram-stained smears of the liver, kidney and bone marrow can be useful diagnostically if treatment has to begin immediately. In smears from tissue, the short rods tend to be more robust and strongly Gram-positive when compared to those made from cultures.

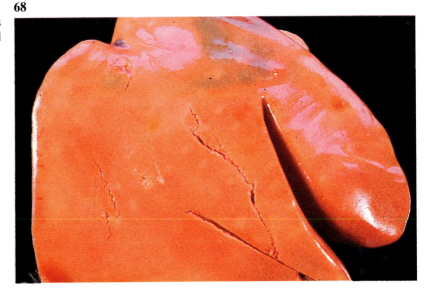

68 The livers of affected turkeys may have a distinctive par-boiled appearance.

69 A clump of *E. rhusiopathiae* in a sinusoid of the liver shown in **68**. The sinusoidal disruption is partly artefactual. Note the hepatocytic vacuolation to the left of the bacteria. This is taken presumptively to indicate fatty change, a hepatocytic feature often observed in septicaemias. Acrylic resin.

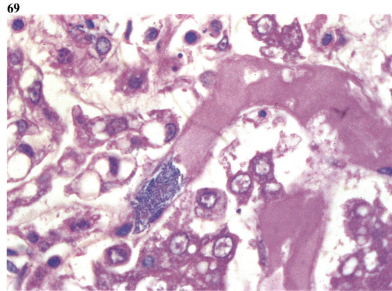

70 Phagocytosis of *E. rhusiopathiae* by Kupffer cells may be a prominent feature of some turkey livers. A section of a pheasant liver is illustrated. Gram.

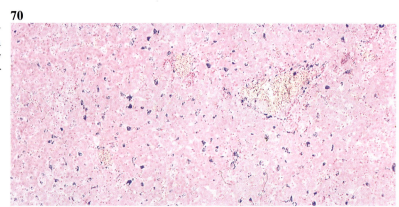

Tuberculosis (*Mycobacterium avium*)

71 The disease is common in free-range fowl but seen only rarely under intensive systems of husbandry. Affected birds gradually become emaciated, and yellowish caseous nodules are most commonly found in the liver, spleen and intestine. Well-developed lesions in the liver can usually be shelled out from the surrounding parenchyma.

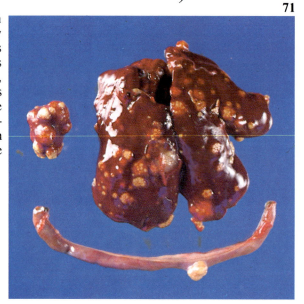

72 A pale granuloma within the marrow cavity of a femur. Lameness often occurs in affected birds due to the development of such lesions, particularly at the distal end of the femur.

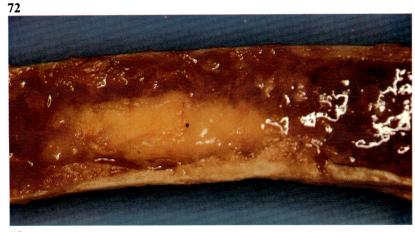

73 Large numbers of acid-fast bacilli are present in smears from most avian lesions. Smears are best made by crushing individual nodules between two glass slides. Ziehl-Neelsen.

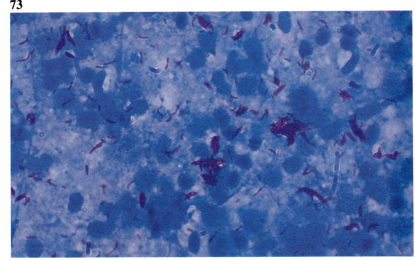

74 Developing tubercle in the liver of a hen. At this stage the central part of the lesion is mainly composed of pale-staining epithelioid cells.

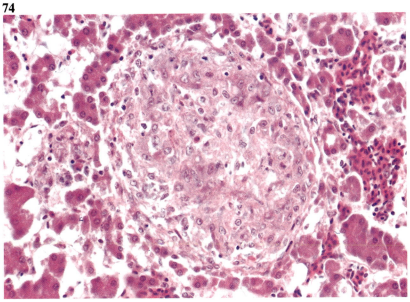

75 A more advanced lesion in which central necrosis has taken place. Giant cells are starting to pallisade round the necrotic zone, and numerous macrophages are present peripherally. Connective tissue encapsulation has not yet occurred.

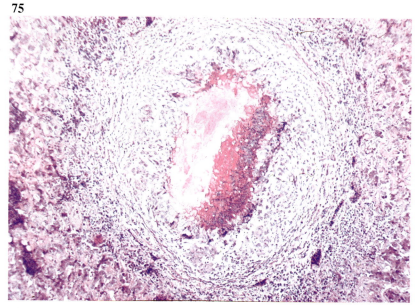

76 A large mass of granulation tissue was present at the thoracic inlet of a commercial layer. Many giant cells were scattered through the lesion, in which there was considerable deposition of amyloid. A giant cell is seen engulfing an amyloid focus.

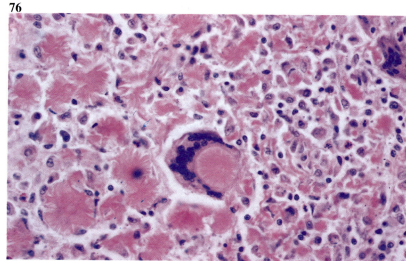

77 A Congo Red stain on the tissue in **76** demonstrates apple-green birefringence of amyloid under polarised light.

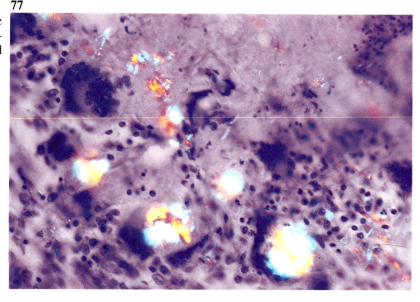

78 Giant cells may be very large. This cell was present in granulation tissue within a peafowl lung.

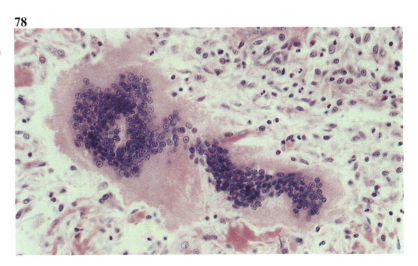

Salmonellosis

This section refers only to diseased birds. Many birds may be infected with salmonellas and show no clinical or post-mortem signs. As used here, the term 'salmonellosis' refers also to the now rare diseases caused by *Salmonella pullorum* and *S. gallinarum*.

79 *S. typhimurium*. Gross lesions are very variable. Heavy mortality may result in young chicks and turkey poults. Focal lesions are present in the liver of this 7-day-old broiler.

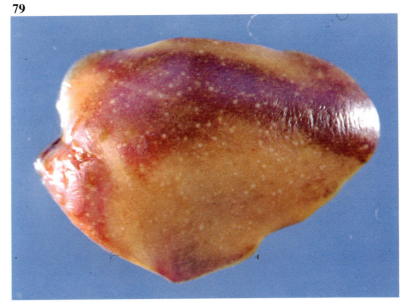

80 *S. typhimurium*. A section of liver from **79**. Necrotic tissue in one of the focal lesions is visible in the lower part of the photograph, and is staining more eosinophically than the unaffected hepatocytes above.

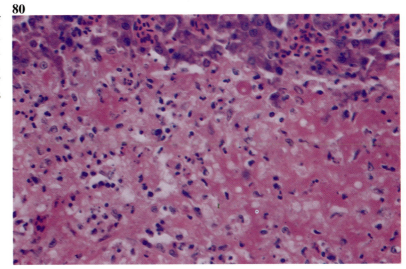

81 *S. typhimurium*. Nervous signs that may appear in infected flocks during the first week of life are usually caused by bacterial meningitis. Acute purulent meningitis in a cerebellar sulcus of a broiler chick.

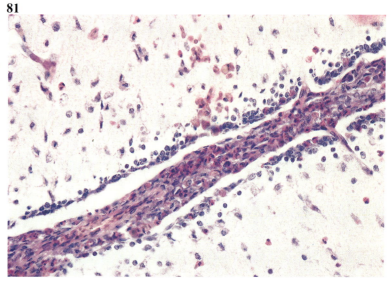

82 *S. typhimurium*. Vermiform appearance of the caeca resulting from acute typhlitis in a 7-day-old broiler. The presence of this lesion is variable and it is not always caused by salmonellosis, but salmonella infection should be suspected when it is seen.

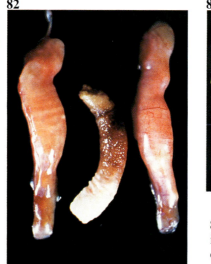

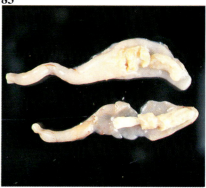

83 *S. typhimurium*. Pale cores of inflammatory debris within the caeca of a broiler chick.

84 *S. typhimurium*. Acute typhlitis in a duckling. Core of eosinophically staining inflammatory debris. Note the thickened mucosa.

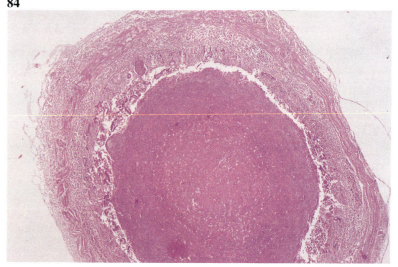

85 *S. typhimurium.* Pericarditis in a 2-week-old broiler. Both pericarditis and perihepatitis (*see* **1**) are sometimes encountered in systemic infections with this serotype and with other salmonellas (e.g. *S. enteritidis*).

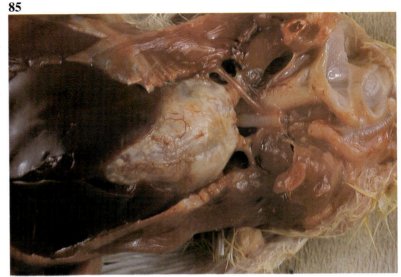

86 *S. gallinarum* (fowl typhoid). In most acute cases the lungs exhibit a brown discoloration.

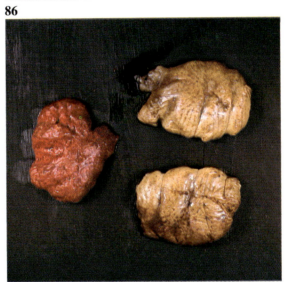

87 *S. gallinarum.* The carcases of birds that have died from the acute disease are jaundiced and the liver on the right displays a characteristic bronzing after exposure to the air. Note also the severe congestion of the spleen.

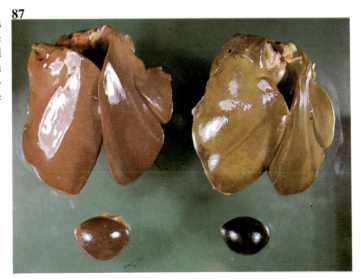

88 *S. gallinarum*. The spleen of this adult fowl is moderately siderotic, probably as a result of a haemolytic anaemia accompanying the disease. Perls'.

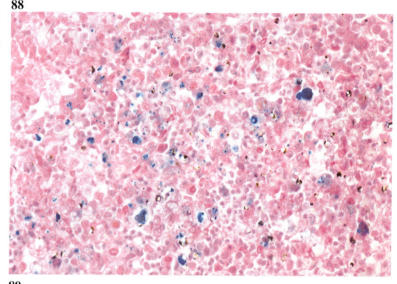

89 *S. pullorum* (bacillary white diarrhoea). Greyish-white necrotic foci in a chick lung. Similar lesions may be present in the heart and liver.

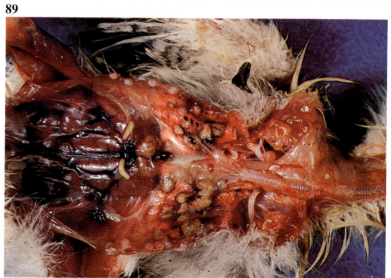

90 *S. pullorum*. Synovitis of hock joints in chicks.

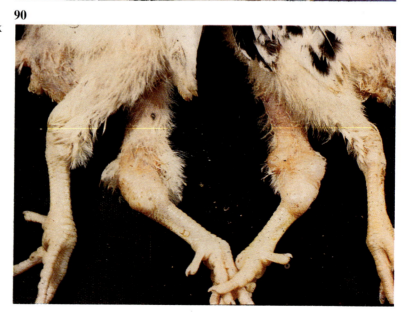

91 *S. pullorum.* Oophoritis is common in adults. This specimen shows a few degenerate ova, some of which are attached to the body of the organ by long stalks. The contents of the affected ova are discoloured and may be inspissated.

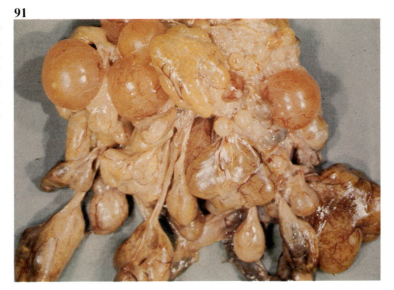

Mycoplasmosis

92 *Mycoplasma gallisepticum.* Swelling of the infraorbital sinuses in a turkey.

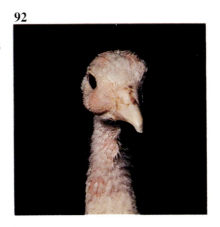

93 *M. gallisepticum.* Infraorbital sinus of a turkey opened to show sticky exudate in an acute case.

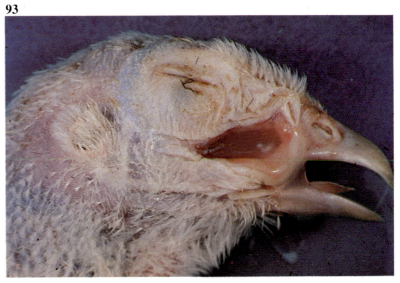

94 *M. gallisepticum*. Gross lesions tend to be more pronounced in the turkey and infection is often accompanied by air sacculitis (yellow pointer) and pneumonia.

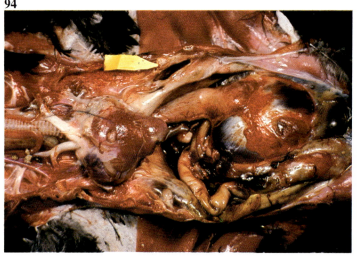

95 *M. gallisepticum*. Pneumonia associated with infection in a turkey. The inflammatory exudate is mixed.

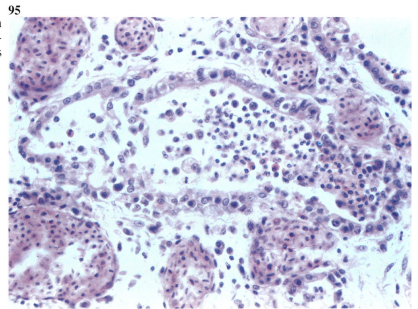

96 *M. synoviae* (infectious synovitis). Subcutaneous bursitis over the sternum in a 9-week-old commercial layer pullet. Note the loss of condition. (N.B. *M. synoviae* may be associated with respiratory disease complexes in broilers; joint and bursal lesions in such flocks are usually absent.)

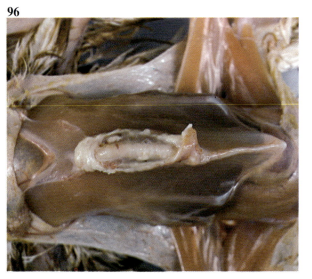

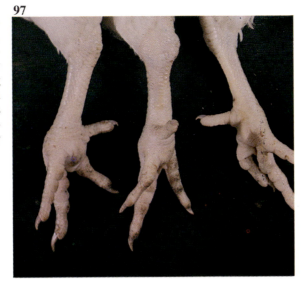

97 *M. synoviae.* Two swollen foot-pads (centre and left) of broilers. This feature may be very pronounced. There is frequently swelling of the hock and main wing joints. As in other mycoplasma infections, egg transmission occurs and the diagnosis should be carefully confirmed, both serologically and culturally.

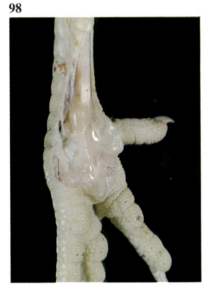

98 *M. synoviae.* Footpad exudate in an acute infection of a commercial layer. The exudate is characteristically glairy and tenacious.

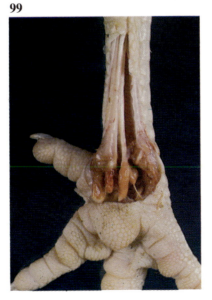

99 *M. synoviae.* Chronic lesions in a footpad of a commercial layer. In chronically inflamed footpads and joints the exudate is often a deep orange-yellow colour.

100 *M. synoviae.* An inflamed
wing joint has been opened to
demonstrate the exudate. Inflammation of wing joints is occasionally seen in staphylococcal
infections, but infectious synovitis
should always be suspected when
lesions are being encountered
frequently in this joint and accompanied by sternal bursitis.

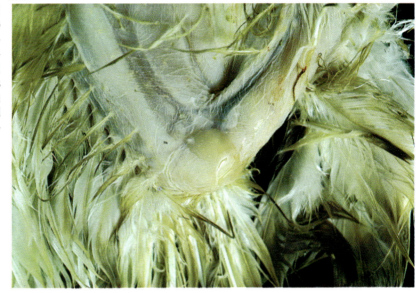

101 *M. synoviae.* Purulent exudate to the right of a chronically
inflamed synovial membrane.

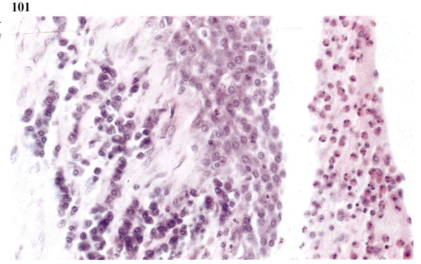

102 *M. synoviae.* The quantity of
joint and bursal exudate may be
greater in turkeys than in fowls. It
also tends to be less glairy and
tenacious. Coagulated exudate is
present alongside the gastrocnemius tendon of a 19-week-old
turkey.

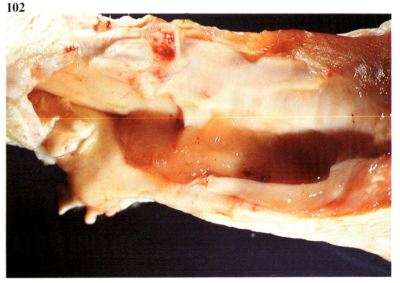

103 *M. meleagridis*. Infection may cause poor growth and feathering, chondrodystrophy, air sacculitis and diarrhoea (turkey syndrome '65). The legs of this turkey have a severe varus deformity at the hock joint.

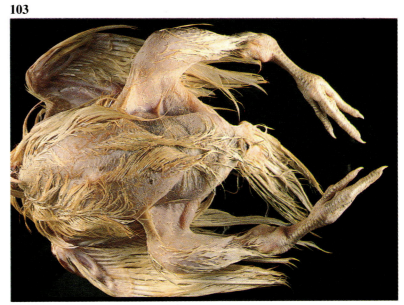

104 *M. meleagridis*. Closer view of a chondrodystrophic tarsometatarsus in the same bird as shown in **103**. Note the shortening and flattening of the proximal head.

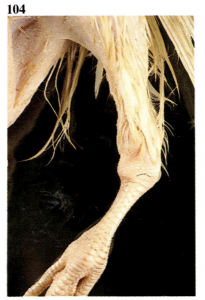

105 *M. meleagridis*. Flecks of caseous exudate within the abdominal air sacs of a 6-week-old turkey.

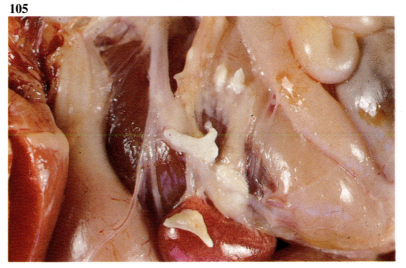

106 *M. meleagridis.* Section of a widened head of an affected tarsometatarsus. Martius scarlet blue.

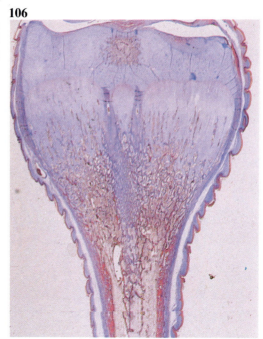

107 *M. meleagridis.* Paucity of developing chondrocytes with some necrosis (arrows) in the transitional zone of the growth plate seen in **106**. Martius scarlet blue.

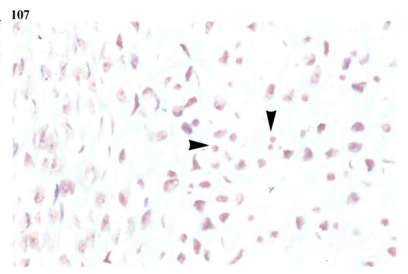

VIRAL DISEASES

Infectious bursal disease (Gumboro disease)

108 Within batches, haemorrhagic lesions are usually encountered in the bursa of Fabricius if mortality is occurring. Lesions vary in severity from a few petechial haemorrhages on the plicae, to a very severe haemorrhage throughout the organ, as seen here. The kidneys of birds that have died are often swollen and pale. This is caused by a terminal dysfunction and is not a nephritis.

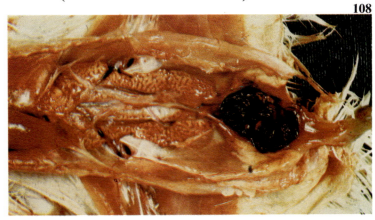

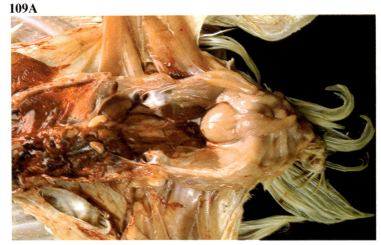

109 The bursa of Fabricius (**109A**) is slightly swollen in a 3-week-old broiler. The small highlight on the surface has been produced by a thin layer of gelatinous oedema covering the serous surface, which is often a prominent feature of the disease. This infection was subclinical. The oedema is more prominent (**109B**) in a fatal case that occurred in another broiler of the same age.

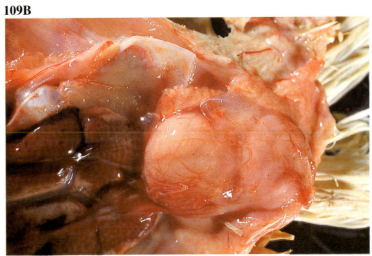

110

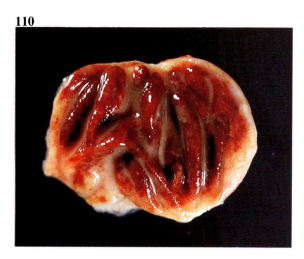

110 Haemorrhagic bursa of Fabricius obtained from a 35-day-old broiler.

111

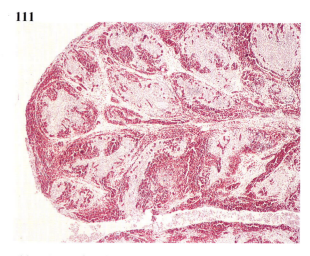

111 Extensive haemorrhages are present in the follicles and interfollicular tissue in this section from **110**. Note the pallor of the follicles, indicating lymphocytic depletion.

112A

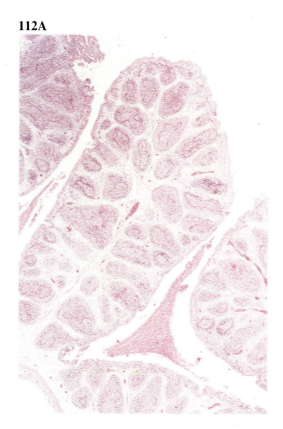

112B

112 Scanning view of affected and unaffected plicae. The extensive lymphocytic loss in this disease results in a much paler-staining section (**112A**) than that found in the unaffected (**112B**) bursa of Fabricius. Visual inspection of the slide or use of a hand lens may therefore raise suspicions of infectious bursal disease.

113 A large mass of purulent exudate in the lumen of the bursa of Fabricius. Note the longitudinal surface indentations in this material caused by the plical folds of the bursa. The kidneys of this broiler are jaundiced, death having resulted from inclusion body hepatitis (*see* **123**). The bursal lesions were caused by an earlier challenge with the infectious bursal disease agent.

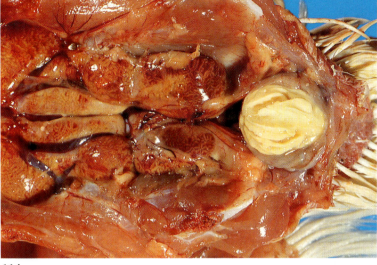

114 Acute inflammation of the bursa of Fabricius in a clinical case. Note the outlines of more darkly staining corticomedullary epithelium (arrows) within an injured follicle. Inflammatory oedema separates the follicles. The interplical space is full of purulent exudate.

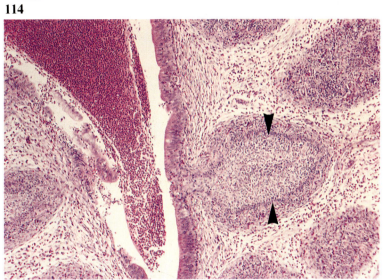

115 Subclinical disease. A higher-power view of an injured follicle reveals lymphocytolysis and heterophilic infiltration. Bursal haemorrhages are absent.

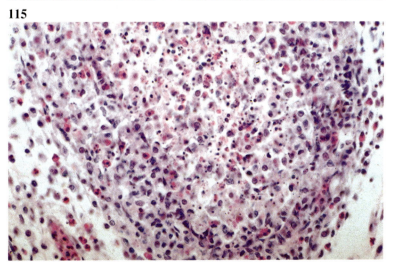

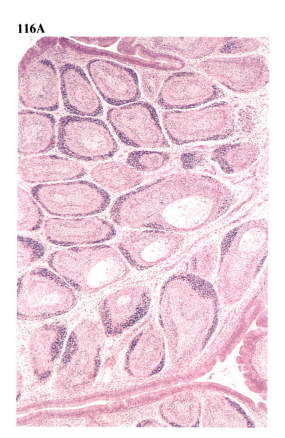

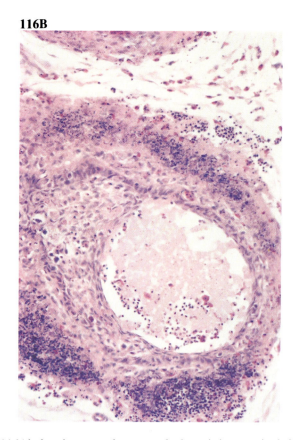

116 Lymphocytic loss has taken place in all follicles (**116A**), but in some there are dark-staining cortical rims caused by the presence of residual lymphocytic nuclear debris. Note the early cyst formation in some central follicles, one such follicle (**116B**) being shown at a higher magnification.

117 Cystic spaces forming in injured follicles may be a prominent feature during resolution. The acute inflammatory reaction is quickly cleared in most cases, leaving severely depleted follicles and fibroplasia of the interfollicular connective tissue. Hyperplasia of the bursal epithelium is often marked at this stage.

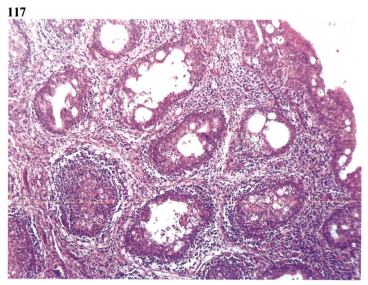

50

118 Linear muscular haemorrhages may be present in birds that have died, particularly on the outside aspect of the thigh. Similar haemorrhages are also observed in breast musculature.

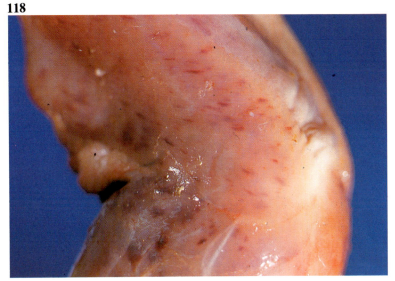

Inclusion body hepatitis

119 The disease is seen mainly in young broilers. The carcases are usually congested, while the macroscopic appearance of the liver varies greatly. Here, an enlarged pale liver contains a few posterior subcapsular haemorrhages. Note the size of the organ compared to the heart.

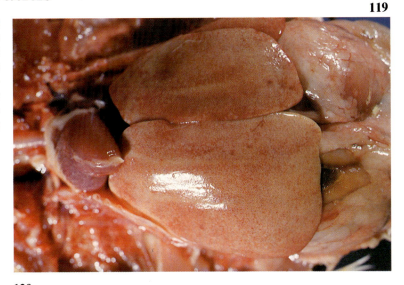

120 Prominent subcapsular haemorrhages in an affected liver lobe.

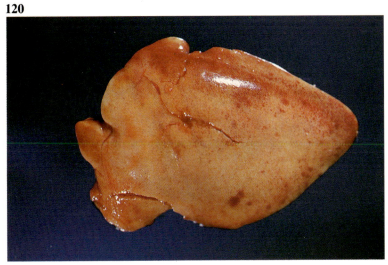

121 Considerable histopathological variation is another feature of this disease. Hepatocytic necrosis may be focal or more diffuse. The appearance of the intranuclear inclusions may range from well-haloed and predominantly eosinophilic bodies (seen here), to large solid basophilic structures (*see* **122**). If lesions are focal, inclusions tend to be seen near their periphery.

121

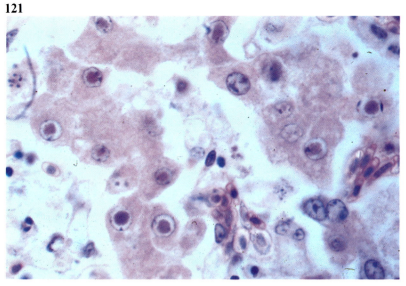

122A

122B

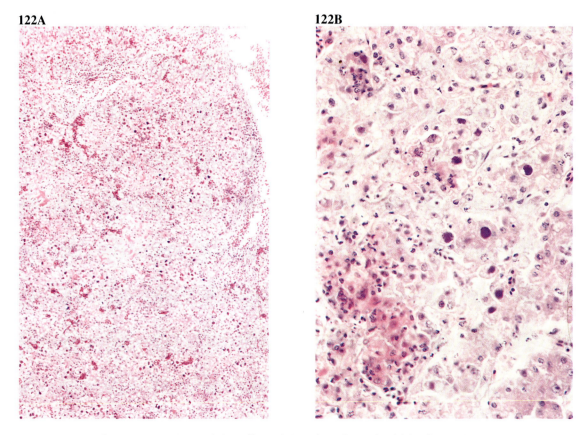

122 Low- and medium-power views of the affected liver in a 2-week-old broiler. The large solid basophilic intranuclear inclusions can be observed as darkly stained dots (**122A**), even on low power.

123 The kidneys are often congested and tinged a muddy yellow colour, probably as a result of jaundice.

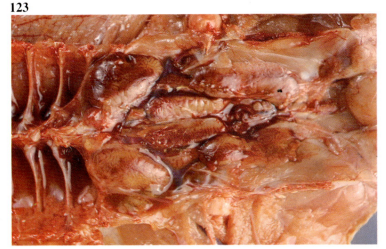

Haemorrhagic enteritis in turkeys

124 Distended small intestine from a turkey grower. Both the distension and the dark colour result from internal haemorrhage. Vent feathers may be blood-stained.

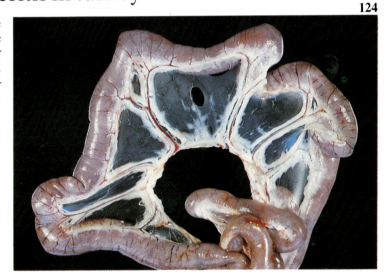

125 An opened small intestine showing haemorrhage and mucosal debris. The extent of the haemorrhage varies considerably.

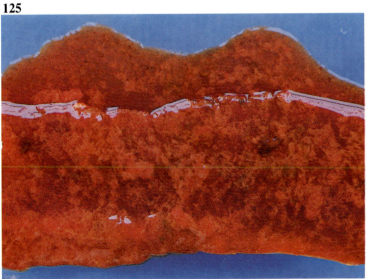

126 Small intestine. There is haemorrhagic disruption of the villi.

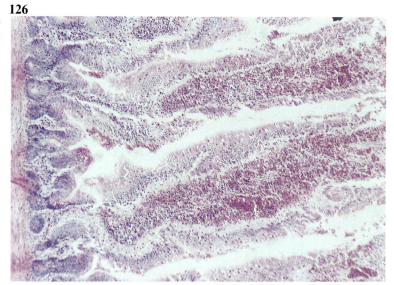

127 The spleens may be swollen and mottled. In pheasants, a group 2 adenovirus related to the haemorrhagic enteritis agent of turkeys causes marble spleen disease, where these splenic features are particularly noticeable. Adult pheasant.

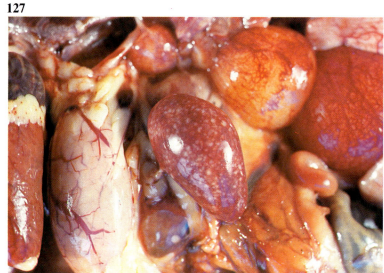

128 The presence of intranuclear inclusions (solid pale-staining bodies are arrowed) within the intestinal lamina propria is a useful diagnostic feature. Acrylic resin.

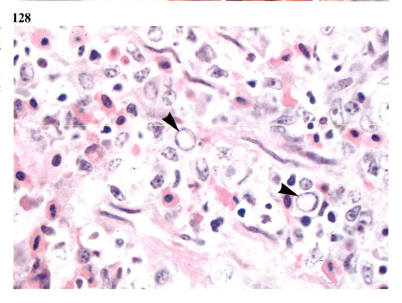

129 Numerous similarly staining intranuclear inclusions (arrows) within the reticulum cells are visible in the spleen. Acrylic resin.

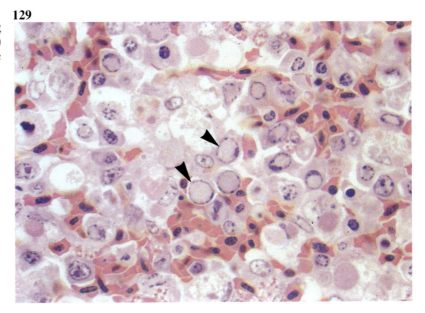

Fowl pox

130 The disease may affect both chickens and turkeys and can cause cutaneous and internal lesions. Here, pox lesions are present in the oropharynx of a hen.

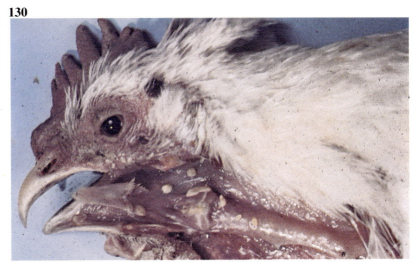

131 Lesions may also occur in the trachea and should be distinguished culturally and histopathologically from diphtheritic forms of infectious laryngotracheitis (*see* **137**). In this cross-section of fixed larynx obtained from a commercial layer, diphtheresis has resulted in almost complete occlusion of the lumen.

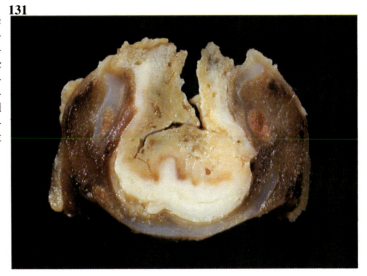

132 Proliferative tracheitis. Masses of intracytoplasmic eosinophilically staining inclusions are visible in the affected epithelium.

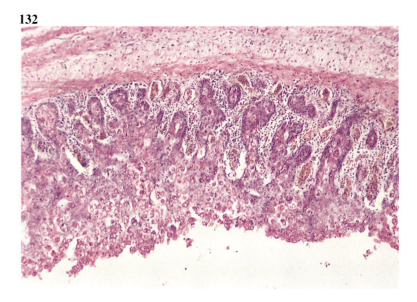

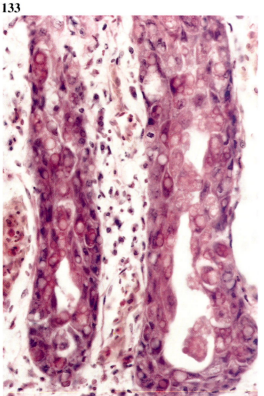

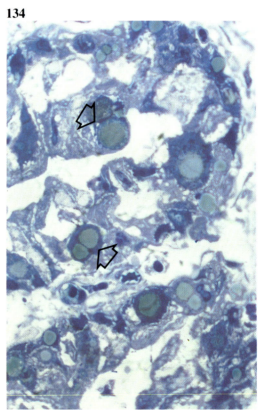

133 Higher-power view of **132**, demonstrating the vacuolar appearance of the eosinophilic inclusions. This is caused by lipid dissolving out of the inclusions during tissue processing, and is a variable feature.

134 Pale-staining lipid globules (arrows) within the cytoplasmic inclusions from **133**. Araldite. Toluidene blue.

Infectious laryngotracheitis

135 Lesions are confined to the respiratory tract. Post-mortem examination may show occlusion of the tracheal lumen with blood and blood clots.

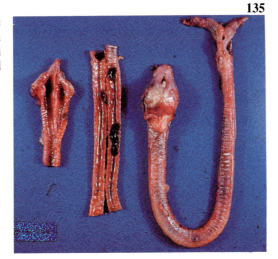

136 Comparison of a blood clot and a fibrinous cast in two tracheas from an outbreak of disease in adult commercial layers. In this incident several of the birds had swallowed expectorated fibrinous casts, which were subsequently found in the crop at post-mortem examination.

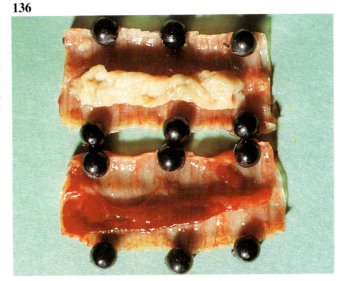

137 In more chronic forms of the disease there may be a pronounced diphtheresis in the trachea.

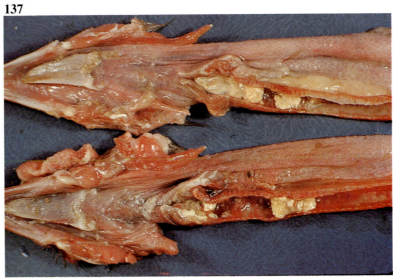

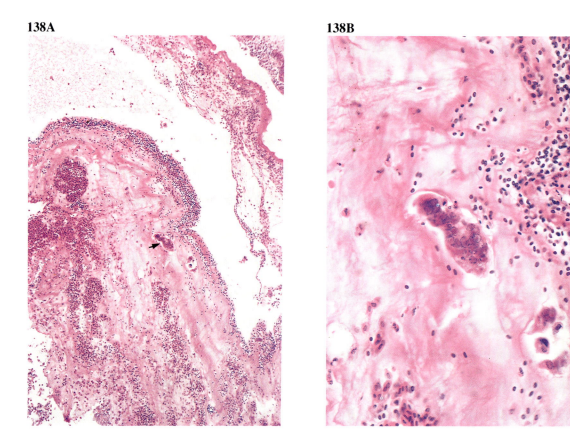

138A

138B

138 Eosinophilic intranuclear inclusions are often best seen in clumps of epithelial cells that have been sloughed from the inflamed tracheal mucosa. Such clumps may be small but often repay close examination. One of these is present (arrow, **138A**) in a mass of sanguinous exudate lying in the tracheal lumen. Higher magnification of the same clump (**138B**) demonstrates typical inclusions.

139 A group of epithelial cell nuclei within a tracheal lumen, demonstrating haloed intranuclear inclusions. If such nuclei are packed a little more closely together than here, the prominent marginated chromatin can impart a 'wire-netting' effect to these clusters, which often catches the eye on histological examination. Acrylic resin.

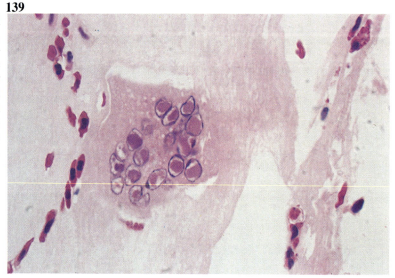

139

Newcastle disease

140 Depending on the strain of virus and its tissue tropism, the post-mortem findings are very variable. Petechial haemorrhages are shown here on the heart and abdominal fat in a congested carcass of a fowl. Haemorrhages on the tracheal mucosa and air sacculitis may be seen with some pneumotropic strains of the virus.

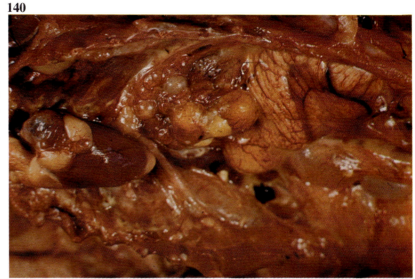

141 If present, proventricular haemorrhages are usually seen on the surface of the papillae and can be distributed in a ring near the junction with the gizzard. Haemorrhagic lesions may also be found in the intestine, particularly on the surface of the caecal tonsils.

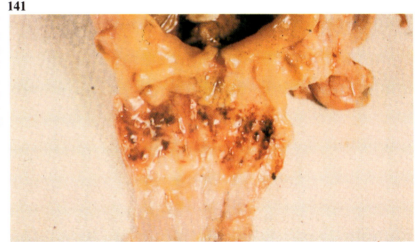

142 Submucosal oedema (arrow) in the trachea of an unvaccinated fowl. Inflammation has resulted in most of the epithelium being shed, leaving small protruding pegs of tunica propria. The lesion is not specific but was observed during outbreaks involving a pneumotropic strain of the virus.

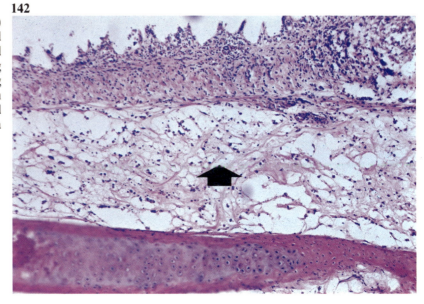

143 Non-purulent encephalitis may be present. In this photograph localised gliosis (arrows) involves the molecular layer of the cerebellum in a fowl.

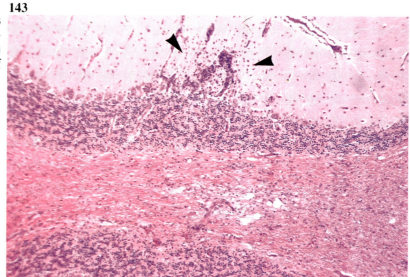

144 Perivascular lymphoid accumulation in a section of cerebrum from a fowl.

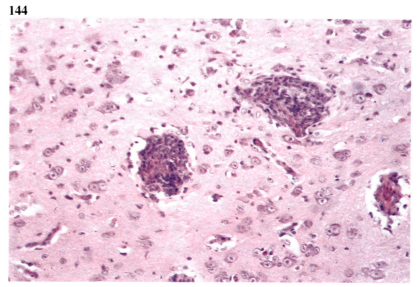

145 Pigeon paramyxovirus. Comparison of pale-shelled and normally pigmented eggs in affected fowl.

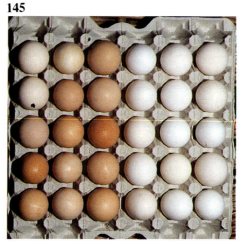

Infectious bronchitis

146 Acute tracheitis in a broiler. Secondary *Escherichia coli* infection is established. Tracheal inflammation may vary from diffuse to a barely perceptible increase in production of a watery mucus. Gross lesions are occasionally confined to the bronchi, and obstruction of these with inspissated inflammatory exudate may result in asphyxiation of the bird.

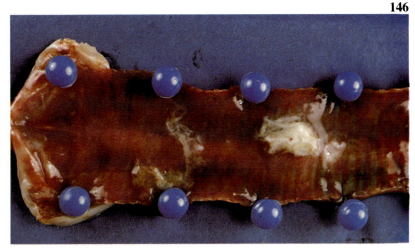

147 A dense lymphocytic infiltration is present in the tracheal mucosa of an unvaccinated 6-week-old broiler breeder. This type of lesion is often seen in field cases but is of doubtful specificity.

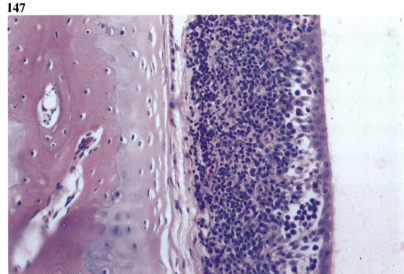

148 Acute nephritis in an unvaccinated 6-week-old broiler breeder. Infectious bronchitis virus was isolated from this tissue. The nephritis was confirmed histologically. The renal swelling and pallor could not be interpreted as a nephritis from the gross appearance alone (*see* **Renal failure**, page 139).

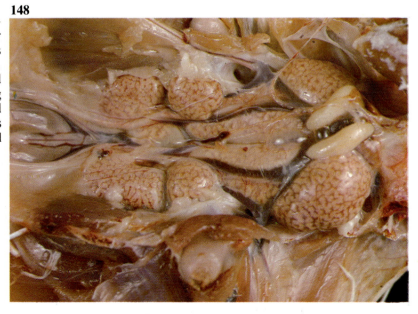

149 Interstitial nephritis produced in an experimental challenge of previously unvaccinated 10-week-old fowls with the H52 strain of the virus. This lesion was characterised by a heavy lymphocytic and plasma cell infiltration. Some plasma cells contain periodic acid-Schiff (PAS)-positive Russell bodies. PAS-haematoxylin.

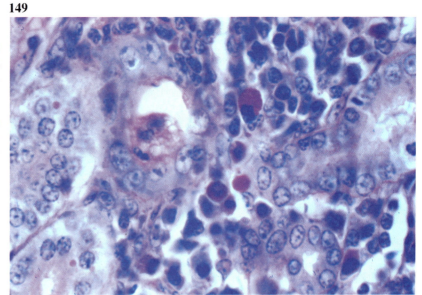

150 A wide range of egg abnormalities may be observed if susceptible laying fowl are infected. Shells are often ridged or have concretions on their surface, or they may be misshapen in other ways, as here.

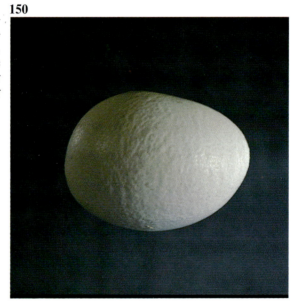

151 The internal quality of eggs may also suffer. Here, the light is being reflected from the outer rim of a watery egg white and there is no internal ring of albumen.

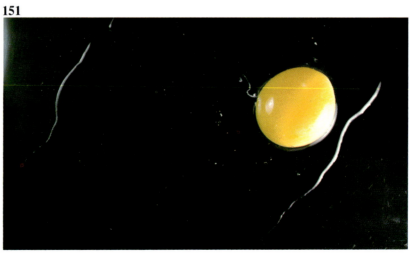

Egg-drop syndrome '76 (127 adenovirus/BC 14 infection)

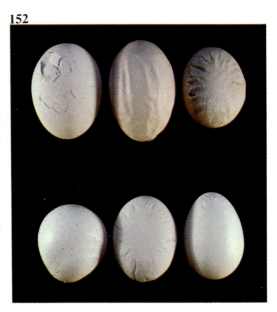

152 This infection is characterised by a drop in egg production or by a failure to peak in laying fowl, either of which may be accompanied by the production of abnormally shelled eggs. These specimens are ridged and irregularly shaped, and some have very thin shells: such features would be difficult to distinguish from some of the shell abnormalities caused by infectious bronchitis. However, soft-shelled and shell-less eggs may also be seen, which features are not usually associated with the latter infection. Diagnosis is best achieved serologically.

Turkey rhinotracheitis

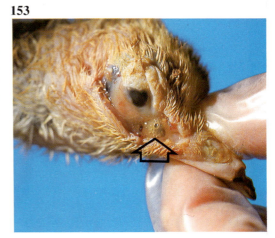

153 Turkey rhinotracheitis in Britain has been associated with primary infection of an agent tentatively identified as a pneumovirus. Clinical signs vary in affected poults and may include coughing, ocular and nasal discharge, submandibular oedema, and swelling of sinuses. In this specimen the infraorbital sinus has been opened to show the presence of mucoid exudate (arrow).

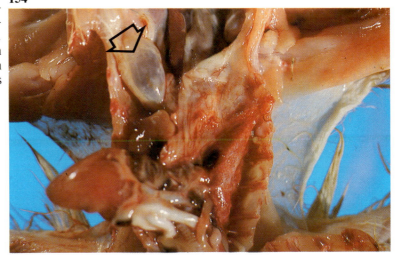

154 Air sacculitis (arrow) was associated with secondary *Escherichia coli* infection in this poult. Such secondary coliform infection is likely to be more severe when the primary viral challenge occurs during the later growing stages.

Chicken anaemia (chicken anaemia agent)

This disease, which is associated with the chicken anaemia agent, has been diagnosed sporadically in Britain. Mortality – usually at 2–3 weeks of age – has largely resulted from secondary bacterial and fungal infections. Such infections tend to be mixed, and post-mortem appearances can vary with the type of organisms present. Gross lesions should therefore be interpreted cautiously; in order to establish a diagnosis it may be necessary to obtain the results of microbiological, immunological, pathological, haematological and epidemiological investigations. Co-infection with the infectious bursal disease agent or other viruses has been reported to enhance the pathogenicity of the chicken anaemia agent.

Figures **155–159** are all of lesions observed in 14-day-old broilers.

155 Pallor of kidneys and skeletal musculature. Such pallor is inconsistent but is usually evident within batches. A patchy dull green discoloration may affect the liver. Secondary staphylococcal infections often give rise to lesions akin to gangrenous dermatitis. Subcutaneous and muscle haemorrhages have also been observed.

155

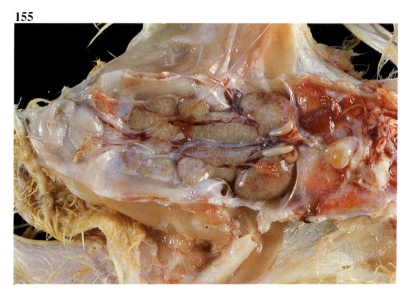

156 The bone marrow in this opened femur is very pale.

156

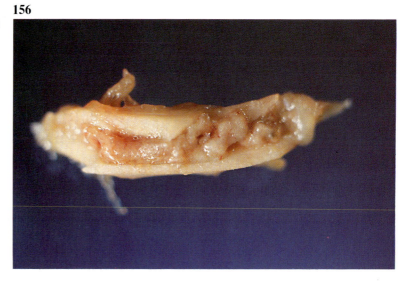

157 A marked depletion of both erythrocytic and granulocytic series is evident in this section of hypoplastic bone marrow.

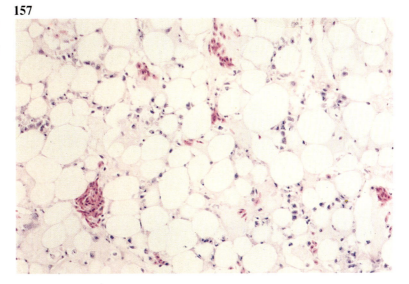

158 Thymic atrophy has resulted in only small lobes (arrows) of the gland remaining. The bursa of Fabricius and the spleen may also be smaller than normal.

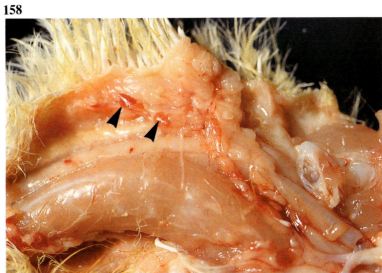

159 A thymic section taken through an atrophied lobe is affected by lymphocytic depletion and lacks corticomedullary distinction.

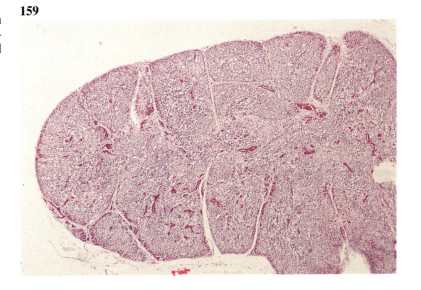

Infectious avian encephalomyelitis (epidemic tremor)

160 Terminal stages may be preceded by ataxia, as in this 14-day-old chick. Muscular tremors may also be detected. Diagnosis is supported by histological examination of the brain, spinal cord, pancreas, proventriculus, gizzard and heart. The disease occasionally occurs in turkeys.

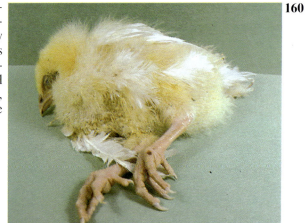

161 A non-purulent encephalomyelitis is widely distributed throughout the spinal cord and brain. Degenerate neurons often exhibit central chromatolysis (arrows). This is not a pathognomonic feature but it can be a useful diagnostic sign, as more neurons show degeneration of this type than is the case in, say, either Marek's disease or Newcastle disease.

161

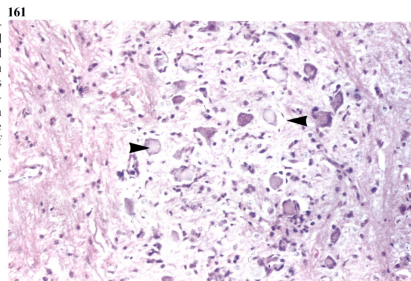

162 A brain-stem neuron undergoing central chromatolysis. The nucleus has moved to the margin of the cell. Note the surrounding gliosis.

162

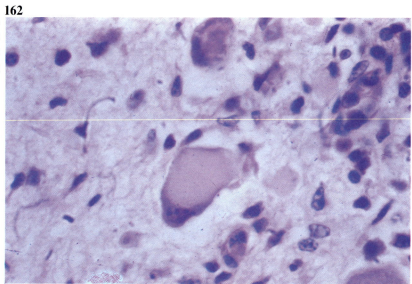

163 Focal gliosis in the molecular layer of the cerebellum in a broiler chick.

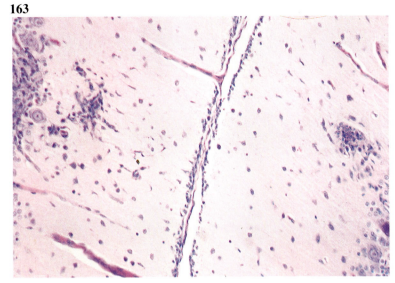

164 Visceral lesions are characterised by the presence of lymphoid infiltration. The pancreas normally contains a few lymphoid foci but in this section there is an increase in their number.

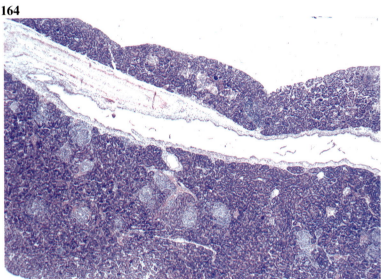

165 Higher-power examination of one of the foci from **164** reveals that it is composed mainly of immature cells.

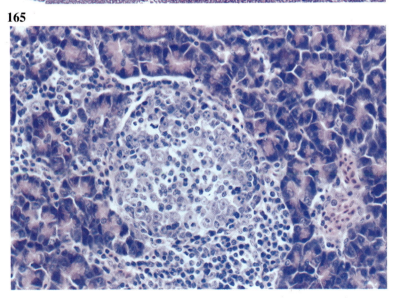

166 Lymphoid infiltration in the proventriculus is restricted to the muscularis. Similar infiltration may occur in the myocardium and in the muscle of the gizzard.

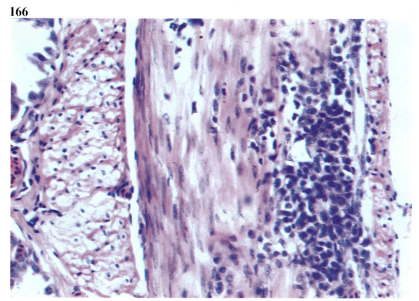

Viral arthritis and tenosynovitis

167 Ruptured gastrocnemius tendon in a broiler, the result of chronic tendinitis. Experimental reovirus infection (*see* **396**).

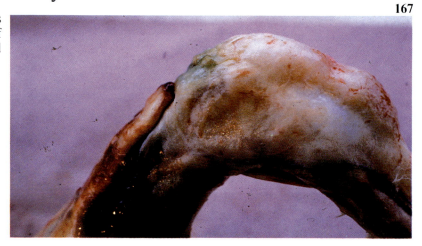

168 Ruptured digital flexor tendons in a broiler. Reovirus was isolated from this field case.

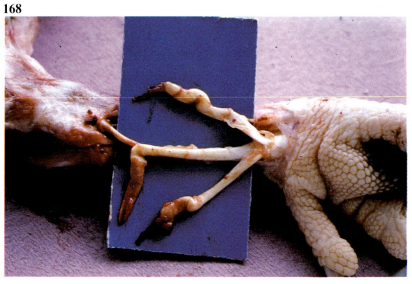

169 Tenosynovitis in a broiler. The tendon sheath is thickened as a result of a non-purulent inflammation involving a dense infiltration of lymphocytes and plasma cells. Experimental reovirus infection.

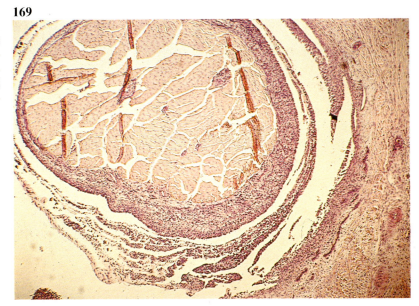

170 Arthritic lesion with pitting of the articular cartilage over the distal tibiotarsal condyles in a broiler. Experimental reovirus infection (*see* **42**).

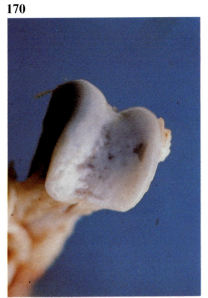

Marek's disease (including transient paralysis)

171 Paresis of the right leg. If both legs are involved, a characteristic posture is often assumed, with one leg pointing forwards and the other held backwards under the body.

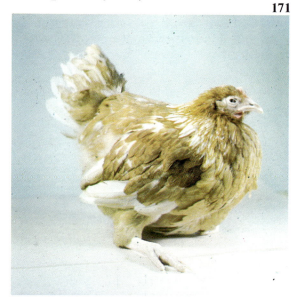

172 This normal sciatic nerve demonstrates the presence of cross striations. These are best seen in daylight rather than under artificial light and are gradually lost as post-mortem changes advance. In Marek's disease, if neural lesions are present, the first appreciable change is a loss of the normal striations together with some focal swelling and yellowing.

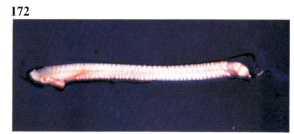

173 One brachial plexus is grossly enlarged. It is important to compare the vagal, brachial, intercostal, mesenteric and sciatic nerves both in the same bird and between individuals within a batch, otherwise slight swelling which may evenly affect most of the peripheral nerves can be missed. There is little doubt about the diagnosis of Marek's disease when gross neural lesions are found. Doubt arises when tumours are present in the absence of peripheral nerve enlargement, when it becomes necessary to examine both the nerves and neo-plastic tissue histologically.

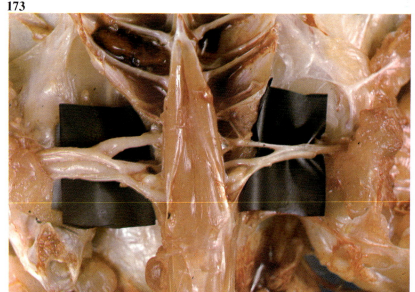

174 Small lymphocytes aggregated around an intraneural capillary. Type C lesion.

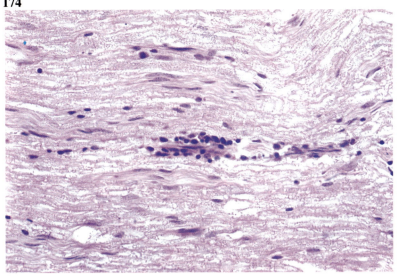

175 Small groups of plasma cells may be present in type B and C lesions. Acrylic resin.

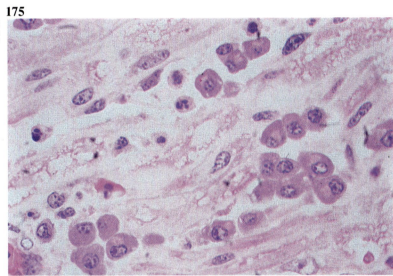

176 An infiltration of small lymphocytes and plasma cells in a peripheral nerve is accompanied by oedema and demyelination. Type B lesion. Acrylic resin.

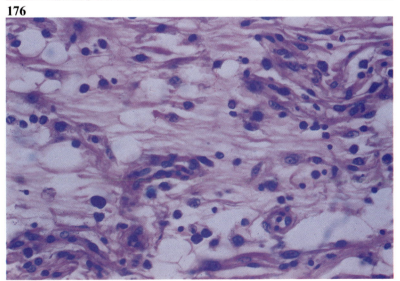

177 Heavy infiltration of proliferating mixed lymphoid cells in a peripheral nerve. Type A lesion.

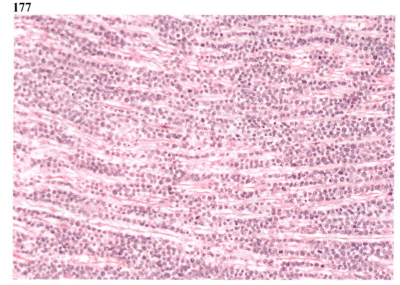

178 Haemorrhage following rupture of the tumorous spleen caused the death of this 6-week-old broiler.

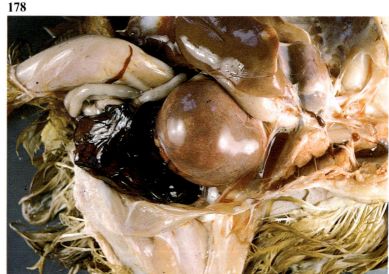

179 Grossly enlarged liver. The organ on the left is diffusely affected; lesions may also be focal. Marek's disease tumours may involve most of the abdominal and thoracic viscera, although the distribution varies considerably. Muscular and proventricular tumours also occur more frequently in this disease than in lymphoid leukosis.

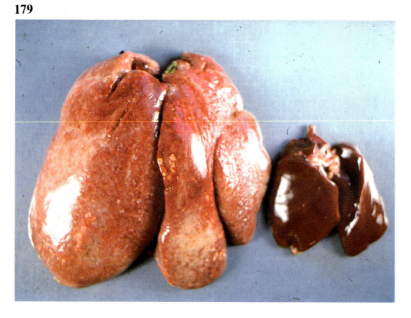

180 The population of neoplastic cells in Marek's disease tumours is nearly always pleomorphic, as demonstrated by this section of skeletal muscle. The large dark-staining cell visible centrally is a so-called 'Marek's disease cell', and is probably a degenerative lymphoblast. Such cells are useful diagnostically but are relatively infrequent.

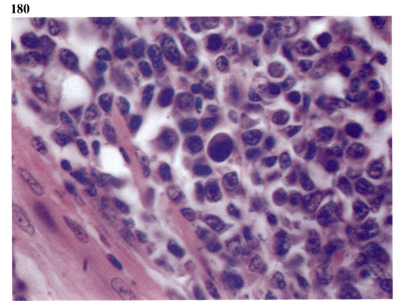

181 Pleomorphic infiltrate in skeletal muscle.

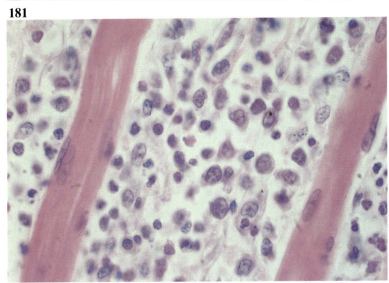

182 The cut surface of this liver demonstrates grey areas of lymphoid infiltration round the portal triads and central veins. This type of infiltration is frequently seen in Marek's disease.

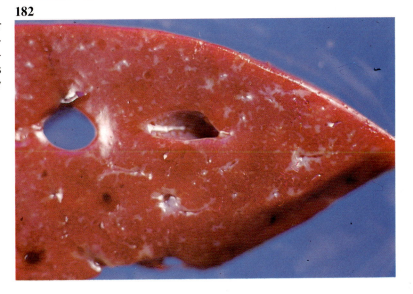

183 Skin tumours are uncommon in Britain but are sometimes encountered in broilers at slaughter. Most of the tumour formation in this specimen is taking place around the feather follicles.

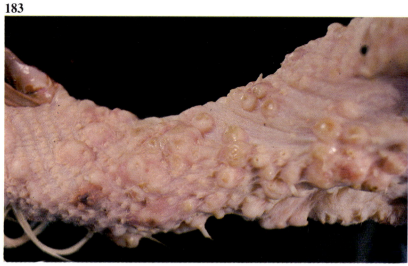

184 This small intestinal villus contains a laminal infiltrate of neoplastic cells. The epithelium on the right is also parasitised with coccidial forms which are similar to those of *Eimeria acervulina*. Concurrent infection with coccidia is often observed in affected birds on deep litter.

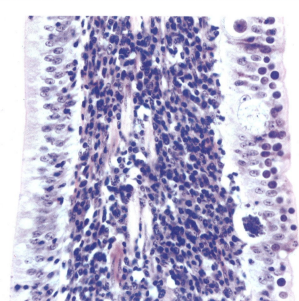

185 An autolysing visceral tumour contains numerous pyknotic nuclei within degenerating neoplastic lymphoid cells. Pyknosis tends to be seen more frequently in autolysing lesions of Marek's disease than in those of lymphoid leukosis (*see* **196**).

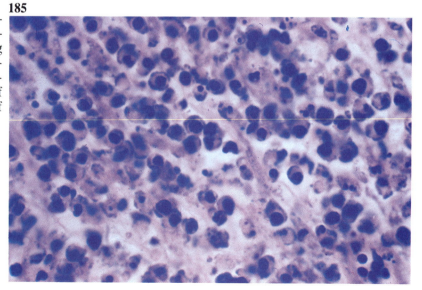

186 Dense perivascular lymphocytic cuffing is a feature of an encephalitis which affects some birds.

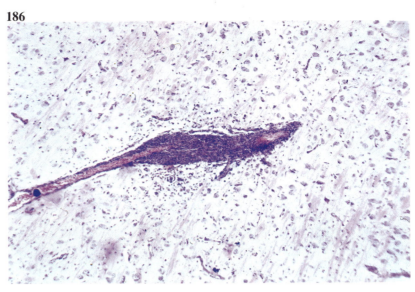

187 Transient paralysis. This pullet shows flaccid paralysis of the neck and tail.

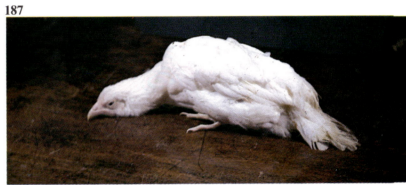

188 A perivascular mononuclear cell cuff in the brain of a bird showing signs of transient paralysis. Note the small cyst-like foci of nuclear debris (arrows).

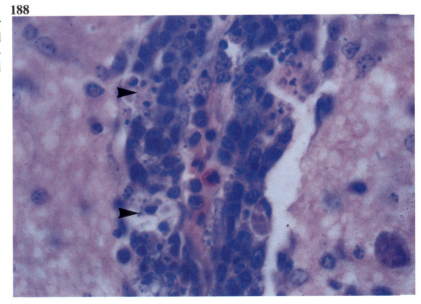

Lymphoid leukosis and other tumours caused by the leukosis/sarcoma group of viruses

189 Lymphoid leukosis. The liver of this adult fowl is greatly enlarged due to the extensive neoplastic infiltration. In the past this disease was often called 'big liver disease'. Although hepatic tumours are frequently found, the macroscopic appearance of the liver cannot be relied on for diagnosis. The size of this liver is, for instance, comparable to that shown in the preceding section on Marek's disease (**179**).

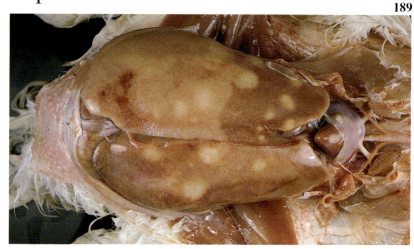

190 Lymphoid leukosis. Lymphoid tumours affecting the kidneys and bursa of Fabricius in the same bird depicted in **189**.

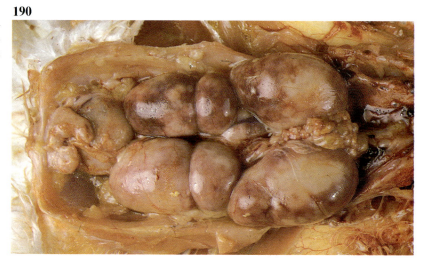

191 Lymphoid leukosis. Tumour formation causing great enlargement of the bursa of Fabricius and focal hepatic lesions in an adult fowl.

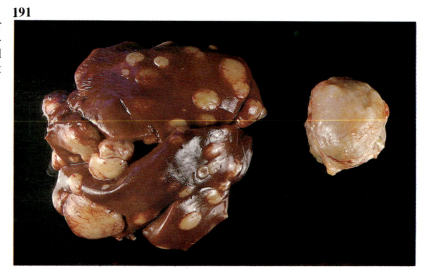

192 Lymphoid leukosis. Expansion of primary intrafollicular tumours in the bursa of Fabricius.

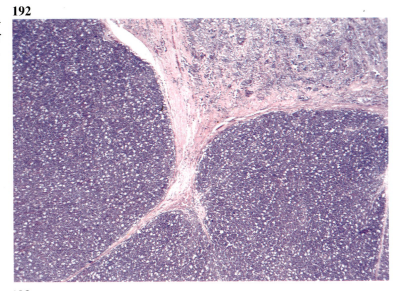

193 Lymphoid leukosis. Tumours are focal and grow by expansion. This contrasts with the more infiltrative lesions of Marek's disease. Here, cords of hepatocytes are being compressed between expanding foci in the liver of a 22-week-old fowl.

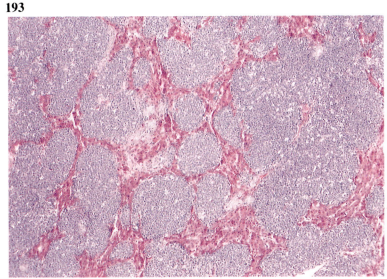

194 Lymphoid leukosis. Tumours are composed of sheets of immature cells which show little or no pleomorphism. Mitoses are moderately frequent in this field.

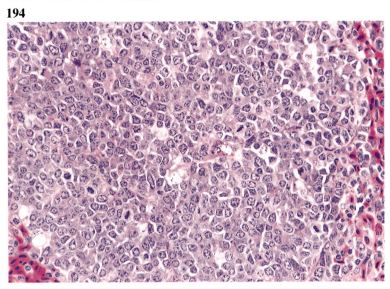

195 Lymphoid leukosis. The nuclei of the neoplastic cells are surrounded by a rim of faintly basophilic cytoplasm and, although not seen here, often contain large violet-staining nucleoli.

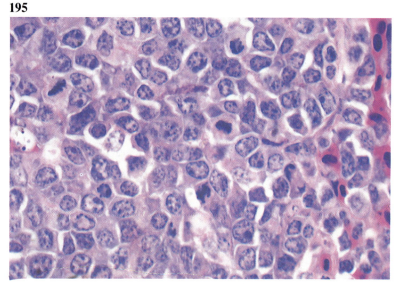

196 Lymphoid leukosis. Many of the tumour cell nuclei undergo karyorrhexis during autolysis (arrows; see **185**).

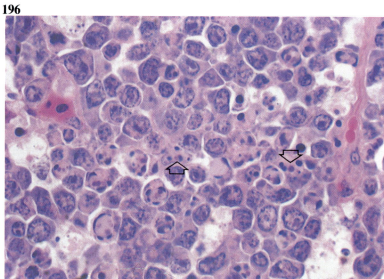

197 Myeloid leukosis. Chalky white myelocytomas are present on the sternum and ribs of this fowl.

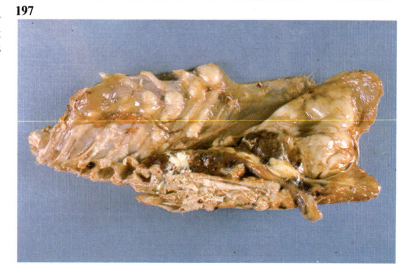

198 Myeloid leukosis. Substernal lesions (arrows) in an adult fowl.

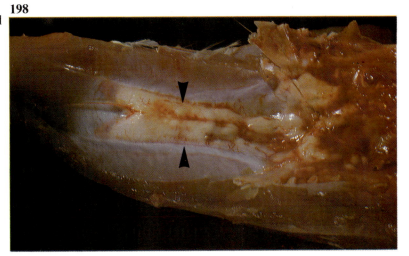

199 Myeloid leukosis. Large numbers of proliferating myelocytes infiltrating skeletal muscle. The eosinophilic cytoplasmic granules are less apparent if the neoplastic infiltrate is composed of myeloblasts.

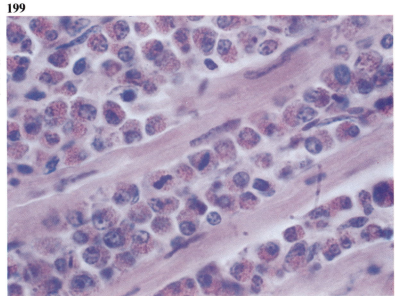

200 Erythroid leukosis. The liver of this fowl is greatly enlarged and cherry red in colour. Similar lesions may occur in the spleen. The disease is rare.

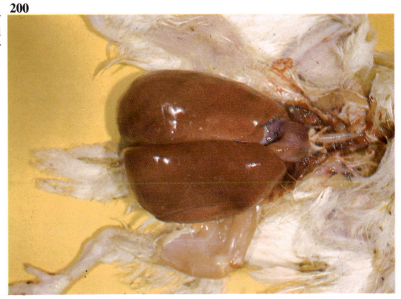

201 Erythroid leukosis. The hepatic sinusoids are packed with basophilic erythroblasts.

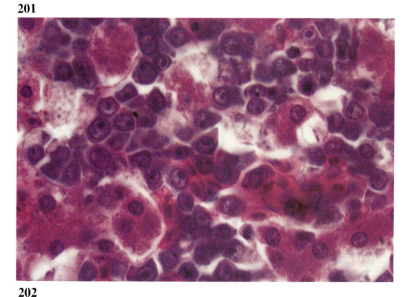

202 Osteopetrosis. This cross-section of an affected tarsometatarsus in a fowl shows the great increase in thickness of the cortical bone.

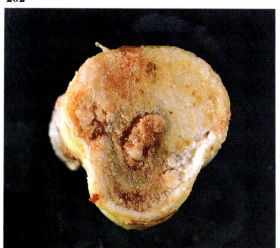

203 Nephroblastoma. This large encapsulated tumour replaced an anterior division of one kidney in a 29-week-old broiler breeder.

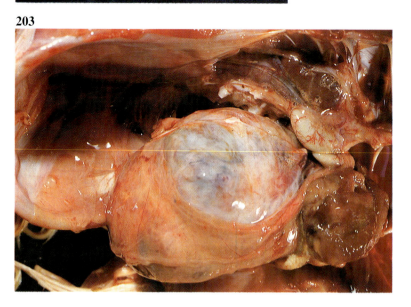

204 Nephroblastoma. Histologically, the tumours are very variable. In this section tubular structures are surrounded by masses of undifferentiated cells. A rim of compressed normal kidney tissue may be present between the developing tumour and the capsule.

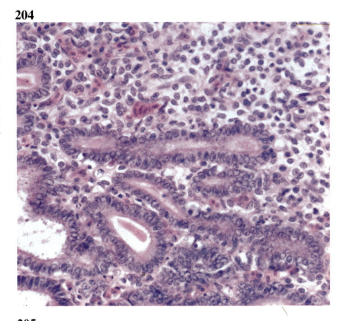

205 Nephroblastoma. Keratinised forms of nephroblastoma are seen from time to time. Large whorls of keratin in this lesion are surrounded by a rim of epithelial cells.

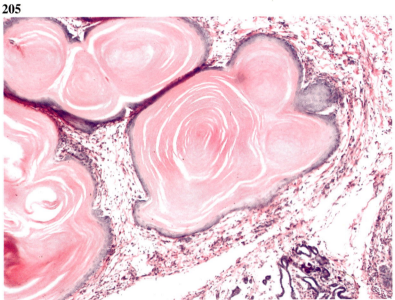

Lymphoproliferative disease of turkeys

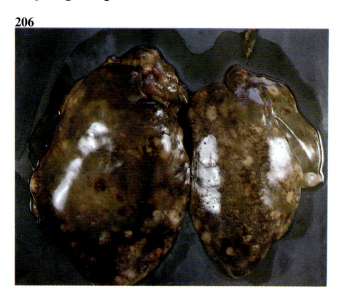

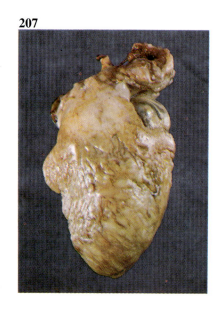

206 Greatly enlarged liver in a 15-week-old grower. This bird also had a *Pseudomonas aeruginosa* septicaemia.

207 Diffuse tumour of the heart.

208 Pale focal lesions in the spleen of a turkey grower. The spleen is often very enlarged in this disease.

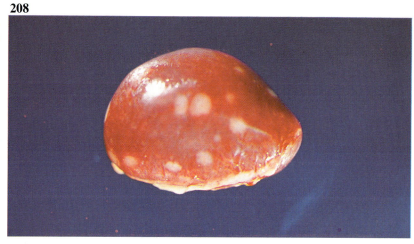

209 Sections of liver showing the pleomorphic nature of the lymphoid tumour.

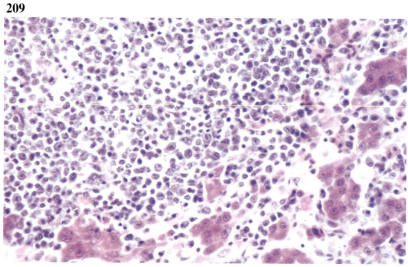

210 The lesion in **209** seen at a higher magnification.

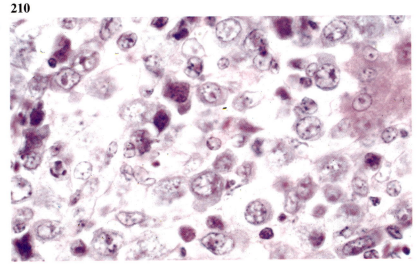

Reticuloendotheliosis virus induced tumours in turkeys

211 Experimental infection. The lesions are focal and grow by expansion. This section demonstrates the population of primitive lymphoblasts.

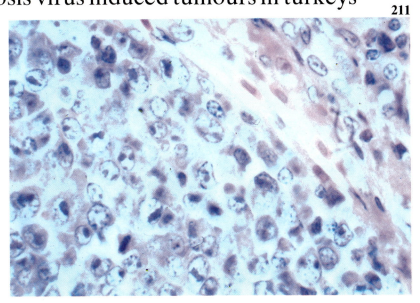

OTHER NEOPLASIAS

Adenocarcinomas of the reproductive tract of the hen

212 Carcinomas may arise in either the ovary or the oviduct. In this specimen the oviduct contains several focal lesions. Early lesions affecting the oviduct may not be seen unless the duct is opened. Occasional outbreaks have been reported.

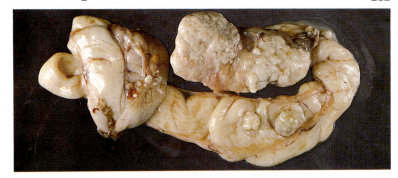

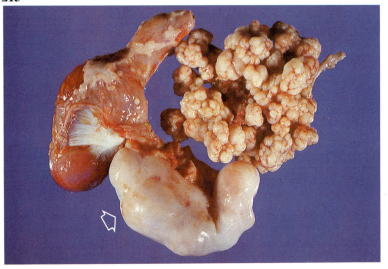

213 Ovarian adenocarcinoma. Adenocarcinoma of the ovary is a common sporadic lesion in adult fowl, particularly in birds over one year of age. The tumour tissue is pale and very firm on palpation. A tumorous ovary is shown together with a grossly thickened duodenum and pancreas (arrow) in a 66-week-old layer (the unaffected gizzard and proventriculus are to the left). Metastasis takes place by trans-coelomic spread and, due to its anatomical position, the duodenal loop is often affected at an early stage in this process.

214 Ovarian adenocarcinoma. Cross-section of the duodenum and pancreas from **213**. Note the small diameter of the duodenum compared to the mass of tumour and connective tissue. The pancreas cannot be distinguished as a separate organ.

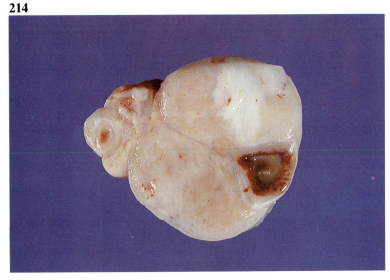

215 Ovarian adenocarcinoma. Rounded metastatic nodules are often implanted on the intestinal mesentery and serous surfaces in the abdominal cavity.

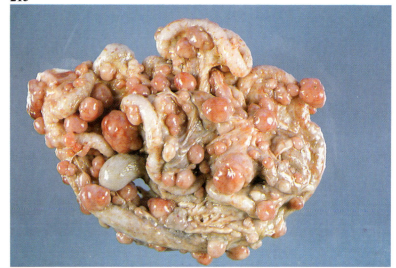

216 Ovarian adenocarcinoma. Most of the metastases are scirrhus in nature due to the proliferation of connective tissue in response to the invading carcinomatous cells.

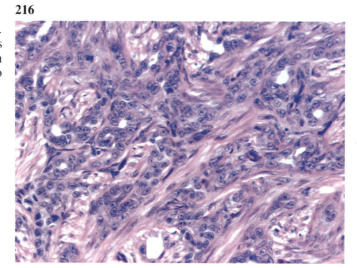

Leiomyoma of the oviduct ligaments

217 These tumours (arrow) are often found in the ventral ligament and are usually composed of both smooth muscle and fibrous elements.

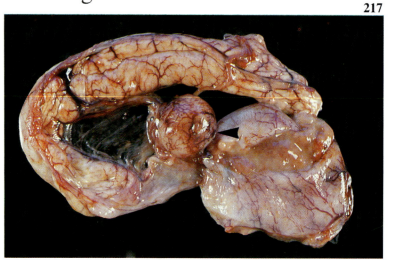

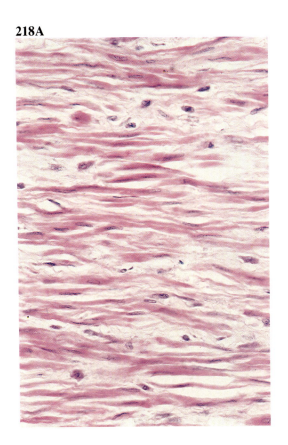

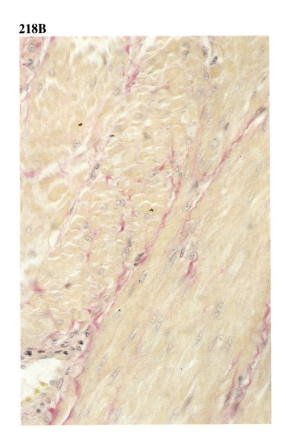

218 A section from a similar lesion to that seen in **217**. Figure **218B** has been stained by the van Gieson method and demonstrates a small quantity of collagen amongst the smooth muscle in the tumour.

Ovarian arrhenoma

219

219 A pedunculated tumour has been cut in half to reveal a large cavernous haemorrhagic area. Rupture of such lesions may lead to fatal intra-abdominal haemorrhage. Virilism may be associated with arrhenomas.

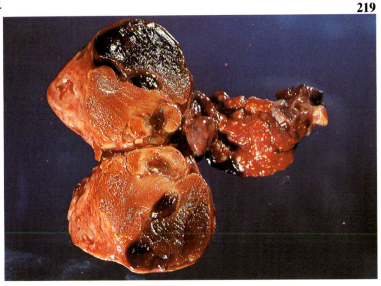

220 Branching cords of epithelium tend to be two cells thick. Both the cells and their nuclei are set transversely to the long axis of the cords. Hyalinisation of the stroma is also evident.

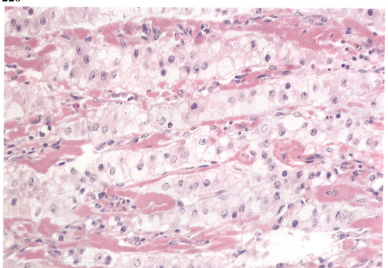

Squamous cell carcinoma of the skin

221 Multiple small crater-like lesions are occasionally found on inspection of broiler carcases at slaughter. Individual ulcers can be seen either side of the midline in this bird but they have coalesced centrally over the whole length of the back. The back and thighs are commonly affected.

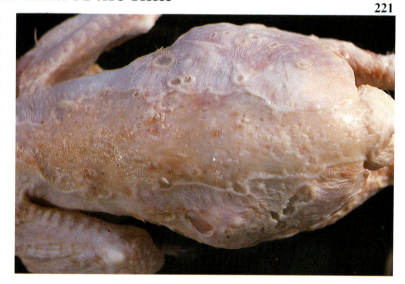

222 Squamous cells invading the dermis from the base of an ulcer. Incipient keratin pearls are arrowed.

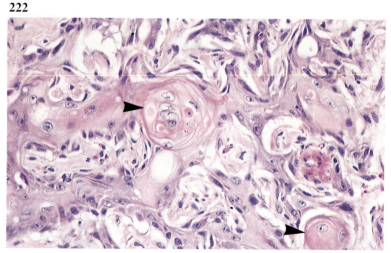

223

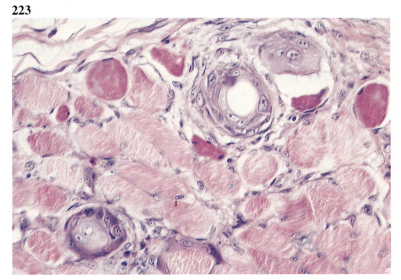

223 Small deposits of tumour cells in the subcutaneous muscle. In spite of such findings the tumour does not appear to metastasize to other tissues during the commercial life of the broiler.

FUNGAL DISEASES

Aspergillosis

224 The disease is common in chicks and turkey poults during the first week or so of life and usually arises from contact with contaminated litter. If the infection is acquired in the hatchery – a rare event these days – pneumonia can develop by 2 days of age. Occasionally, lesions are confined to the bronchi and are not observed unless the lung is cut through. The miliary lesions seen here are in the lung of a 9-week-old pheasant.

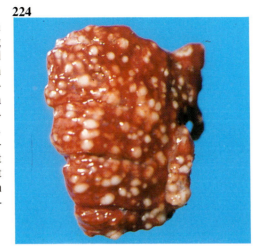

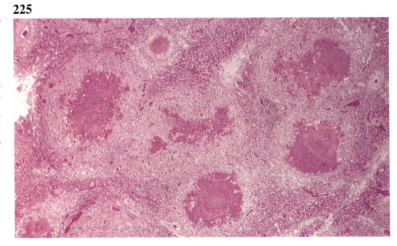

225 The miliary lesions consist of rapidly developing granulomas. In this turkey poult the rounded pulmonary masses comprise central zones of inflammatory debris and fungal hyphae; at this early stage they are surrounded by a pale rim of macrophages amongst which giant cells are starting to form. Acrylic resin.

226 Concentric inflammatory zones within a nodule attached to the intestinal serosal surface in a chick.

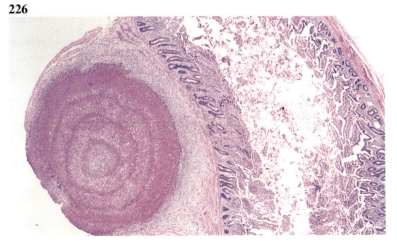

227 Basophilic septate branching hyphae of *Aspergillus fumigatus* within a pulmonary nodule in a chick.

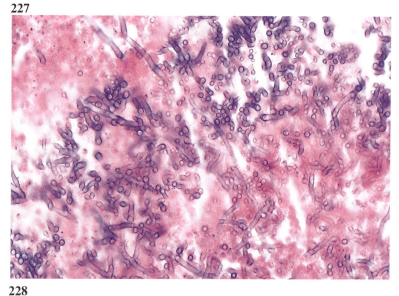

228 Necrotic tissue is quickly removed by giant-cell activity. In this section hyphae are protruding through a ring of giant cells. PAS-haematoxylin.

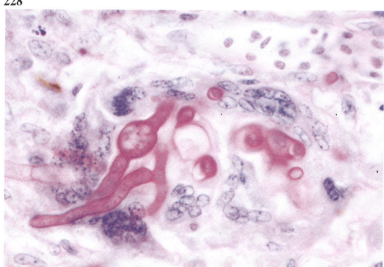

229 Infections in chicks and turkey poults often result in the development of small nodules on the surface of the thoracic and abdominal air sacs. These lesions have a concentric appearance and a depressed centre. Later growing stages in the turkey may be affected by an air sacculitis in which there are much larger plaques of purulent material present.

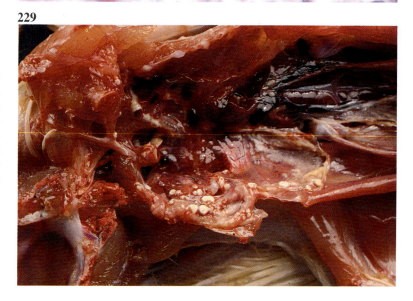

230 Heavy pulmonary infections in young birds may lead to focal encephalitis. Small hyphae in the brain stem of a turkey poult are surrounded by an intense inflammatory reaction and some attempt at early giant-cell formation. PAS-haematoxylin.

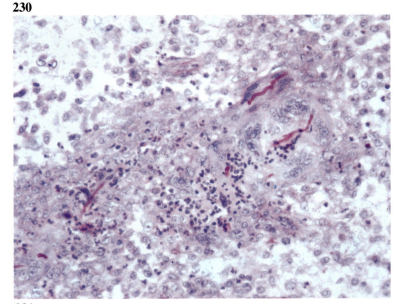

231 Conidiophores are sometimes seen if pulmonary lesions extend into an air space.

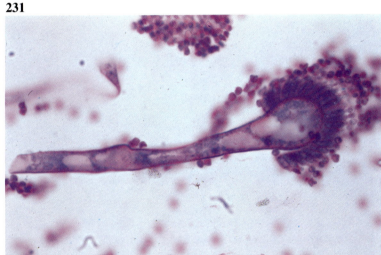

Dactylariosis

232 Occasional outbreaks may result in severe losses in both chicks and poults. *Dactylaria gallopava*, introduced as a contaminant on bark litter, caused heavy mortality in broilers on the farm from which this specimen was obtained. Pulmonary lesions were minimal but severe cerebellar and brain-stem lesions led to an outbreak of disease which clinically resembled encephalomalacia. The infection has destroyed most of the posterior folia. PAS-haematoxylin.

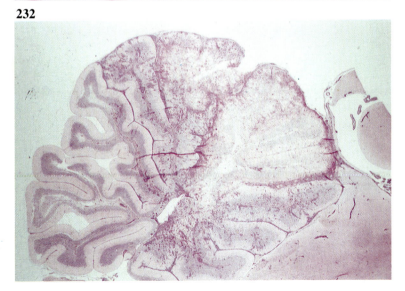

233 Higher magnification of **232** reveals slender hyphae ensheathed by newly formed giant cells. PAS-haematoxylin.

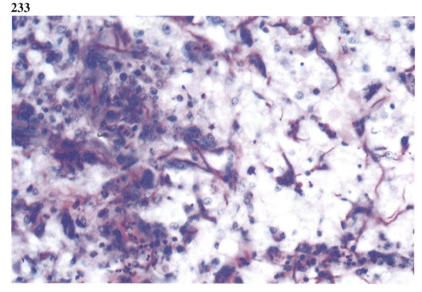

234 Young colonies of *D. gallopava* growing on Sabouraud's medium after 48 hours' growth at 42°C.

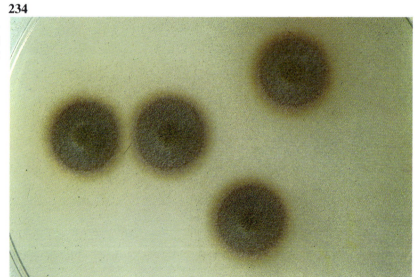

Candidiasis

235 A heavy deposit of desquamated epithelial cells provides the typical 'Turkish towelling' appearance in the crop of a turkey. *Candida albicans* infection.

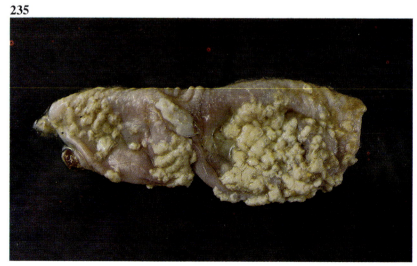

236A

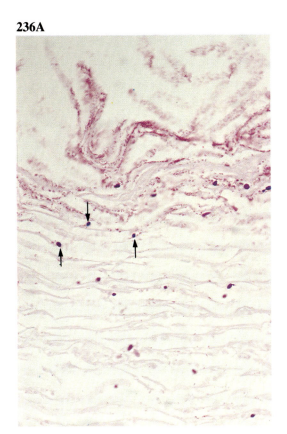

236B

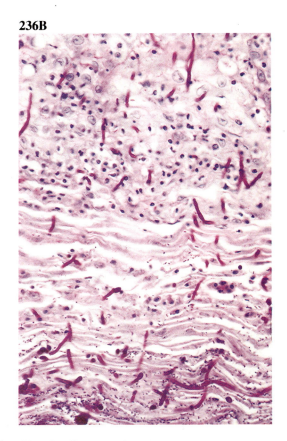

236 An affected crop in a 10-day-old turkey poult stained by the Gram and PAS methods. Note that a few yeast cells are Gram-positive (arrows, **236A**) but that the pseudohyphae have not taken up the stain in this preparation. Compare with a PAS-stained section (**236B**) from the same tissue in which both stain positively.

237 Most of the fungal growth in the crop takes place in the superficial mass of detached cells, but some invasion of intact epithelium usually occurs. The pseudohyphae are poorly demonstrated with haematoxylin and eosin but are strongly positive to PAS and other fungal stains. PAS-haematoxylin.

237

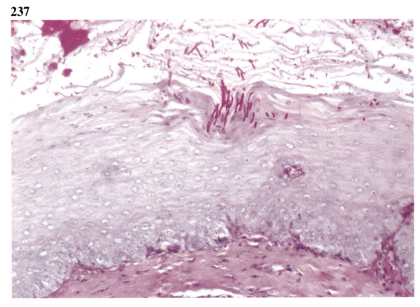

238 Pseudohyphae within crop epithelium. PAS-haematoxylin.

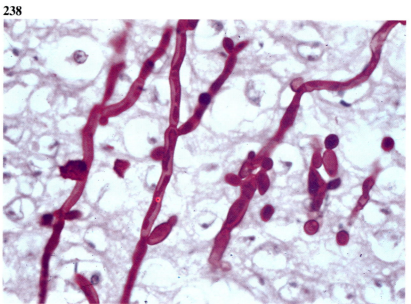

PARASITIC DISEASES

Ascaridiasis

239 The heavy infestation with *Ascaridia galli* shown here is not common under intensive systems of husbandry, except in the presence of a disease such as Marek's. Light-to-moderate worm burdens are encountered more frequently.

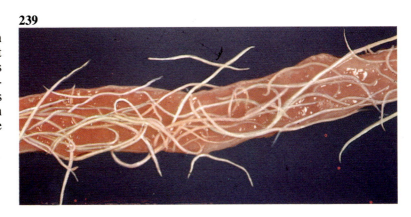

Capillariasis

240 Infestation of the small intestine may have a marked effect on egg production in fowls maintained on deep litter. The affected bowel is usually pale and distended with fluid contents, while the mucosa is slightly roughened. The worms are difficult to see in the intestine with the naked eye but are readily visible in smears. Yellow bi-operculate eggs are seen here in a worm obtained from a racing pigeon.

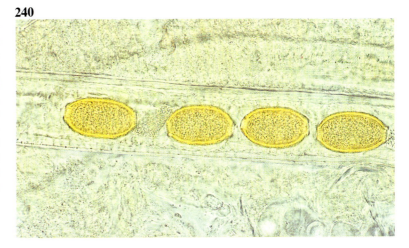

241 Capillaria worms seen in cross-section and attached to the small intestinal mucosa of a racing pigeon.

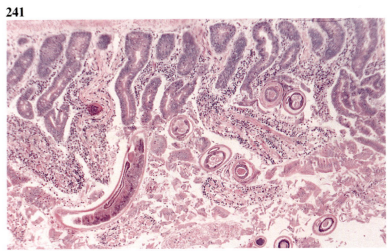

242 Infections of the crop are occasionally found in turkeys. There is a marked thickening of the mucosa. Cross-sections of two worms and a central cluster of eggs are illustrated.

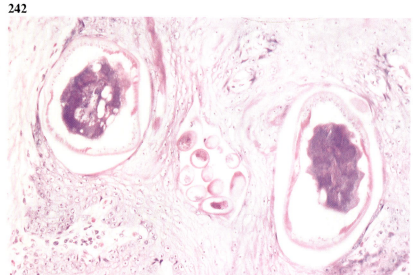

Coccidiosis

243 *Eimeria tenella.* Caeca of a young pullet distended with blood.

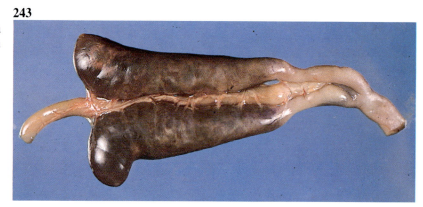

244 *E. tenella.* Extreme pallor of the pectoral muscles as a result of caecal haemorrhage.

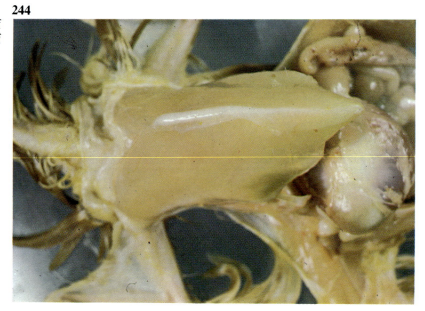

245 *E. tenella*. Caeca opened to show haemorrhagic debris. There may be firm caecal cores in sub-acute cases or in birds that are recovering. These are not usually adherent to the mucosa and, depending on how long they have been present, their gross appearance does not always betray their haemorrhagic origin.

245

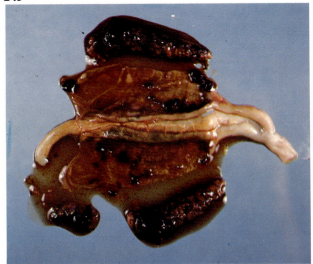

246 *E. tenella*. Smears of the haemorrhagic mucosa will demonstrate the large second-stage schizonts. These are best viewed under a fairly low illumination of the microscope stage. A solitary oocyst is also present near the centre of this field.

246

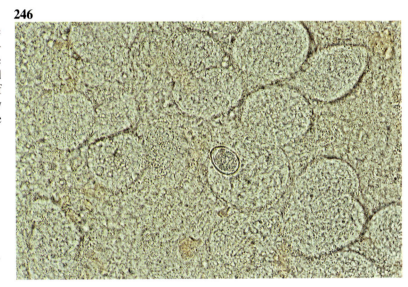

247 *E. tenella*. Second-stage schizonts (containing merozoites) in disrupted caecal mucosa.

247

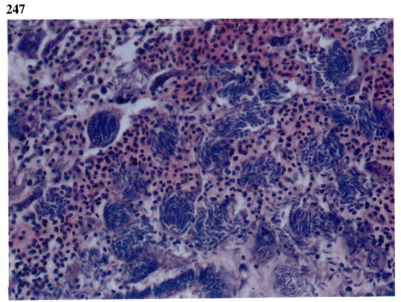

248 *E. tenella*. A large number of oocysts in a caecal core from a partly healed lesion.

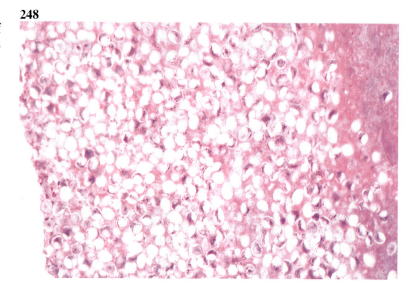

249 *E. necatrix*. Distended small intestine showing mottled haemorrhages through the serous surface.

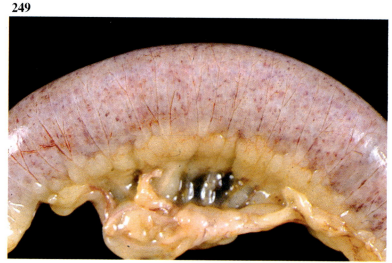

250 *E. necatrix*. Opened intestine from **249**. The lumen is full of mucoid debris. Mucosal smears show similar second-stage schizonts to those observed in *E. tenella* infestations.

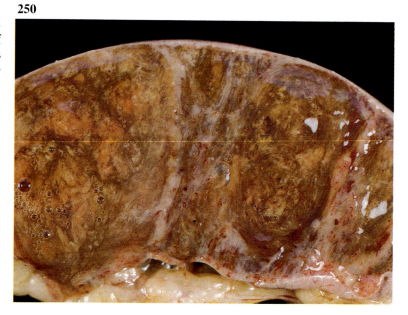

251 *E. necatrix*. Large blood clot in the small intestine of a laying fowl.

251

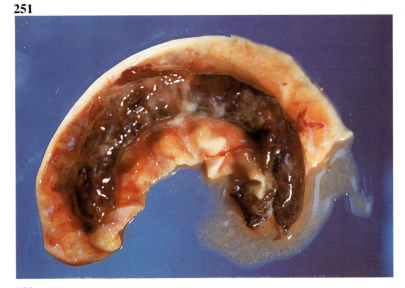

252 *E. necatrix*. Oocysts are found in the caecum and, in this photograph, are distending a crypt.

252

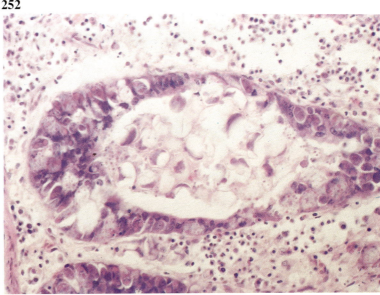

253 *E. maxima*. Small intestinal mucus is often orange-brown in colour.

253

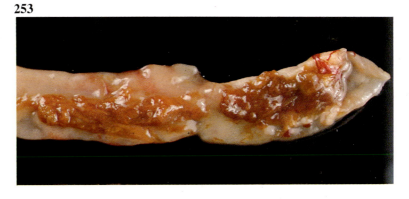

254 *E. acervulina.* The mucosal surface of this intestine is roughened and slightly congested. The affected broiler breeder had concurrent lesions of Marek's disease. Small transverse white flecks can often be seen from the serous surface.

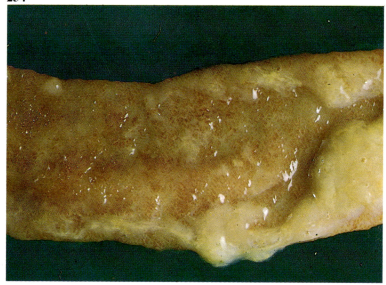

255 *E. acervulina.* Densely parasitised small intestinal epithelium.

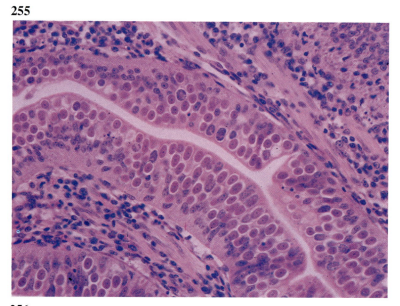

256 *E. brunetti.* Sloughing of small intestinal mucosa in a 7-week-old broiler breeder. The presence of oocysts in smears distinguishes this lesion from uncomplicated cases of necrotic enteritis (*see* **55**).

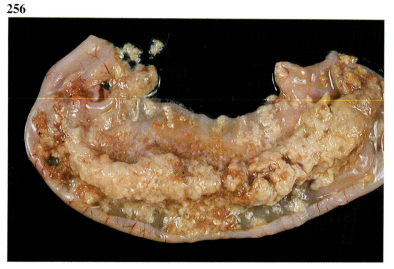

257 *E. brunetti.* Necrosis extending through the depth of the intestinal mucosa and also involving the muscularis in a 3-week-old broiler breeder. A few oocysts (arrows) are present. Heavy growths of *Clostridium perfringens* are usually isolated from such lesions. Secondary bacterial hepatitis is common.

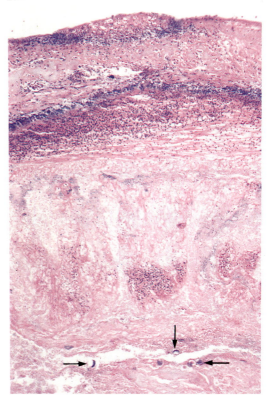

258 *E. meleagrimitis.* The small intestine of this turkey poult is distended with pale fluid contents.

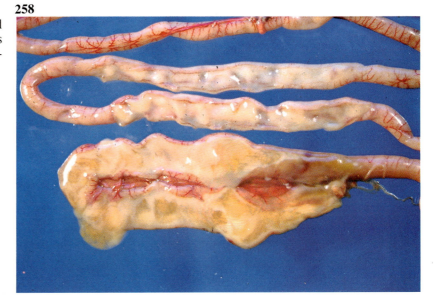

Histomoniasis (*Histomonas meleagridis*)

259 The disease is now a rarity in turkeys except in small flocks that have access to ground used by chickens; it occurs occasionally in the fowl. These specimens were obtained from 15-week-old commercial pullet replacements being reared on deep litter. The liver is studded with lesions that have dark centres and pale rims. The caeca are distended with cores of inflammatory debris that were firmly adherent to the mucosa. Localised peritonitis over the caeca is common in the turkey.

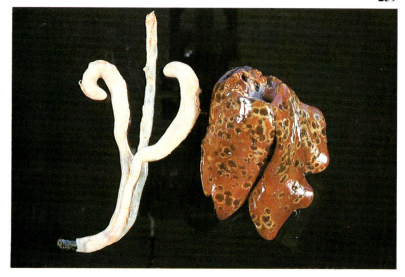

260 Cross-section of an affected caecum from **259**. The pale central core is adherent to the mucosa. The muscularis is invaded by the parasites.

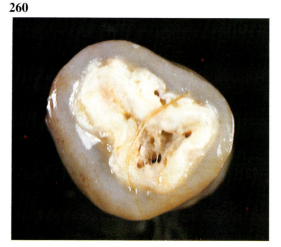

261 Numerous rounded PAS-positive parasites in a liver section from **259**. Note the artefactual contraction of each histomonad from the boundary of the host tissue. The parasites are often difficult to identify in chronic lesions. The presence of rounded spaces containing no stainable material and set within an inflammatory response should raise suspicions and lead to a careful histological search for still-intact parasites. PAS-haematoxylin.

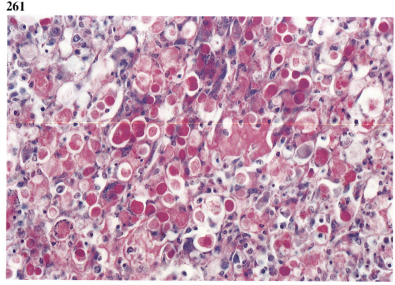

Cryptosporidiosis

262 The small basophilically staining parasites are present on the surface of the luminal epithelium in the bursa of Fabricius in a broiler. The epithelium is hyperplastic. Similar lesions may be observed in the trachea. No clinical signs were shown in this case but respiratory disease has been reported in both turkeys and broilers. The small size of these organisms makes them difficult to see. They stain strongly with PAS.

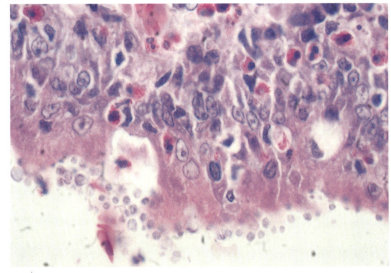

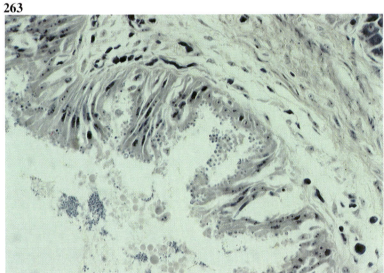

263 Cryptosporidia have also been identified in the urinary tract of some avian species. A parasitised ureteral branch of a jungle fowl is illustrated. This infection was presumed to have ascended from the cloaca. Haidenhain's iron haematoxylin.

Scaly leg

264 The presence of the parasite *Knemidocoptes mutans* has caused the leg scales of a bantam to become raised due to the accumulation of debris underneath.

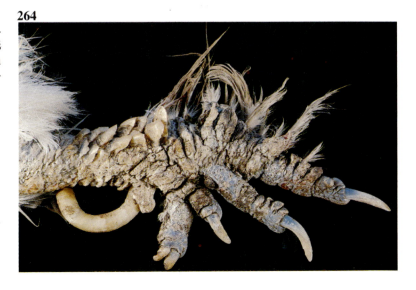

Lice

265 Large numbers of eggs (species unidentified) on feathers of a laying fowl from a flock where egg production was poor.

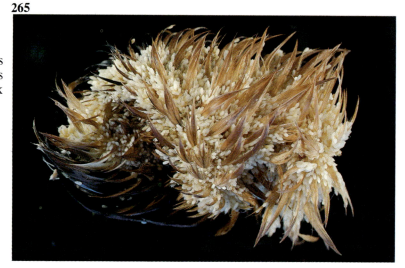

Red mite (*Dermanyssus gallinae*)

266 Small dark mites on the roof of the mouth in an adult broiler breeder. This bird had died as a result of a severe anaemia caused by the parasite. As the mites feed at night but otherwise live off the host, they are not usually found on the skin surface; the upper digestive tract of anaemic birds should therefore be searched for the parasite if the loss of blood cannot be otherwise explained.

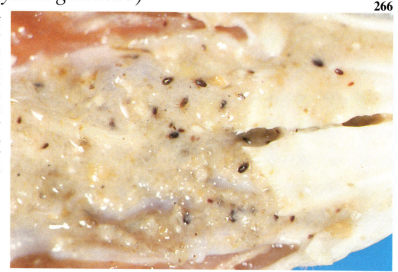

267 The presence of red mite should be suspected in layers if egg production falls and anaemic birds are submitted for examination. Note the red colour of those mites that have recently fed. The mites are shown at about 10 times life size.

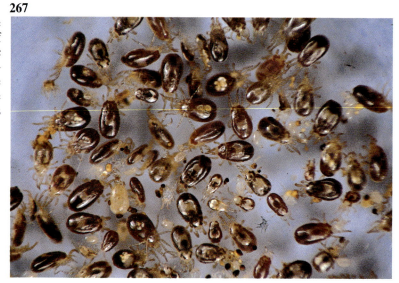

Northern fowl mite (*Ornithonyssus sylviarum*)

268 These live continuously upon the birds, and are seen here on the feathers of a broiler breeder that was submitted with excoriated tail and vent skin. The mites move quickly and are easily transferred to the gloves and arms of the person doing the post-mortem examination.

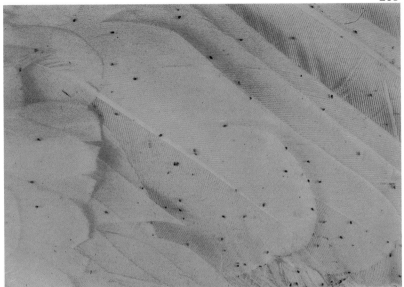

NUTRITIONAL DEFICIENCIES AND METABOLIC DISORDERS

Riboflavin deficiency

269 Clubbed down may occur in the unhatched embryos and day-old chicks from parent flocks that receive inadequate levels of this vitamin.

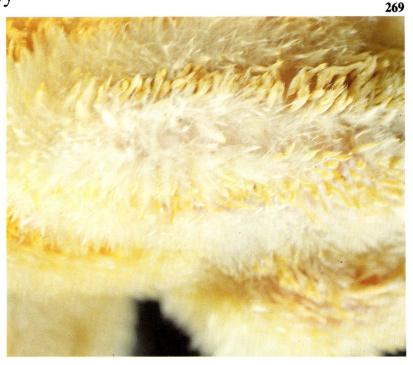

270 Curled toe paralysis. Young chicks may develop clinical signs at about 10–14 days of age if they have been eating a deficient ration. The birds remain alert but are unable to rise from their hocks. They exhibit a flaccid paralysis and an in-curling of the toes (**270A**), which is not maintained after death. Recovery takes place rapidly after treatment. The same chick is shown (**270B**) after receiving a multivitamin preparation in the drinking water for 48 hours.

270A

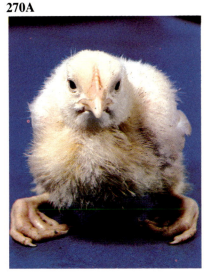

270B

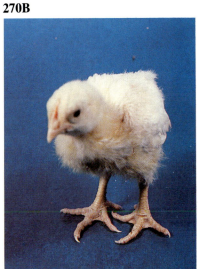

271 The sciatic nerves are swollen and may be discoloured. There is a slight surface oedema in this specimen.

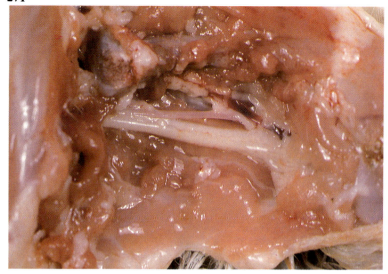

272 Schwann cell proliferation (arrow) is visible in this section of a sciatic nerve taken from a broiler chick with curled toe paralysis.

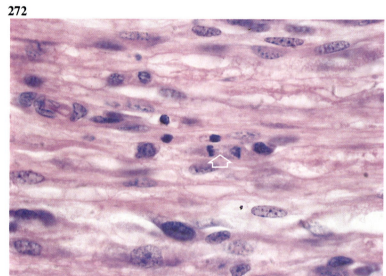
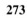

Encephalomalacia

273 Opisthotonos in a 5-week-old replacement pullet. Clinical signs are most often seen between 2 and 3 weeks of age if chicks or turkey poults have been on a ration that is deficient in vitamin E or from which they are unable to obtain a sufficient amount of the vitamin.

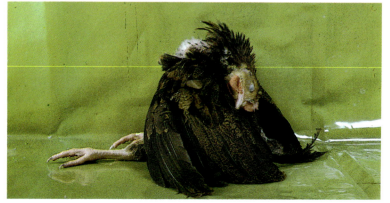

274 Haemorrhage within a partly fixed cerebellum of a 2-week-old turkey poult. When present, gross lesions vary from extensive haemorrhage of the cerebellum to a barely detectable oedema and flattening of the cerebellar gyri and of the cerebral hemispheres.

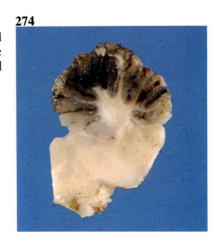

275 Cerebellar haemorrhages. Haemorrhage usually occurs in severe lesions but is not always present.

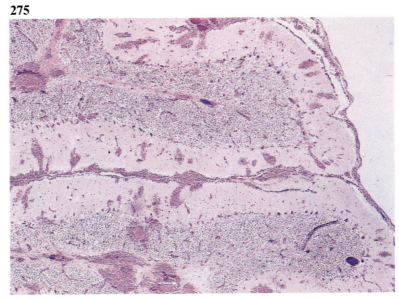

276 Focal malacic lesion in a cerebellar medullary ray. The lesions are most frequently observed in the cerebellum and brain stem, but can affect other parts of the brain, too. They are usually obvious in sections but a slight focal pallor may also be an indication of early change, which is best appreciated via a low-power examination or by the use of a hand lens.

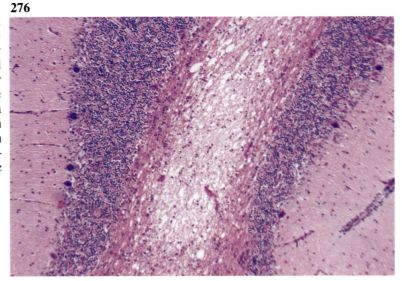

277 Hyaline capillary thrombi are often associated with the malacic lesions. They should be carefully searched for in suspicious cases. Martius scarlet blue.

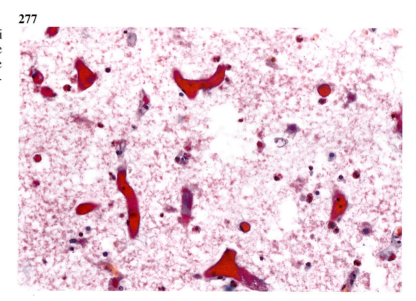

278 In Britain, nervous signs are sometimes seen in young chicks, typically at 4–7 days of age, resulting from well-defined malacic lesions that are mainly distributed in the brain stem (arrow) and cerebrum. Such disease may be transitory in the flock. The cause of these incidents and possible relationship, if any, to the disease observed at 2–3 weeks of age is uncertain. Hyaline capillary thrombi are present in the lesions.

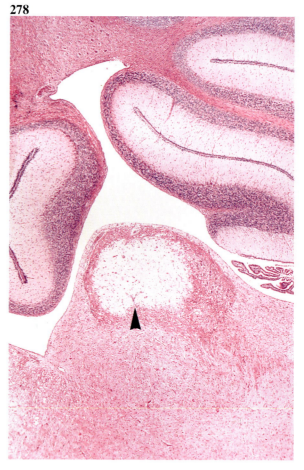

279 Distribution of lesions in the brain stem of a 4-day-old chick affected by the syndrome described under **278**. Note the sparing of the cerebellum. Weil's.

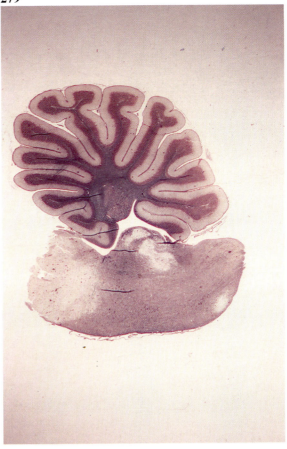

Hypovitaminosis A

280 Squamous metaplasia in the oesophageal mucous glands (arrows) of an adult layer has resulted in great distension of the glands with keratin. Acrylic resin.

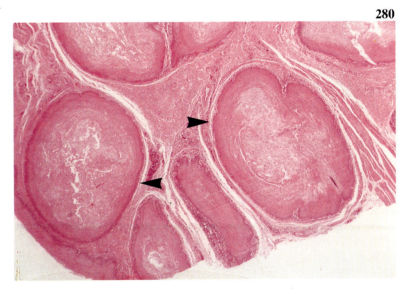

Rickets

281 Rickety rosary in a 3-week-old chick. Field outbreaks appear to occur more frequently in turkey poults. The disease is usually caused by a deficiency of vitamin D_3 but may also be produced by a lack of calcium or phosphorus or by an imbalance of these two minerals. An inability to rise from the hocks and severe depression are the principal clinical signs.

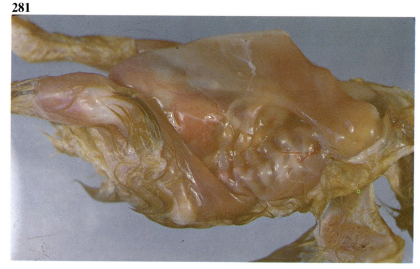

282 Beading of the rib heads is a common feature.

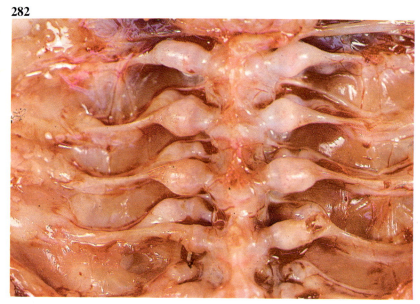

283 Post-mortem assessment of bone strength may be difficult in any bird under 2 weeks of age, but in rickets the tarsometatarsi are usually rubbery and do not break cleanly under pressure. Displacing the beak also provides a good indication of the strength of the facial bones.

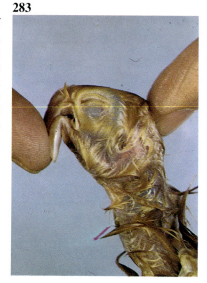

284 The histopathology of rickets varies with the aetiology. It may be difficult, however, in some field cases clearly to distinguish the cause microscopically. In deficiencies of calcium or vitamin D₃ the zone of proliferation in the physeal cartilage tends to be thickened and there is a narrower zone of hypertrophied cartilage. This section demonstrates poor penetration by metaphyseal blood vessels into the hypertrophied cartilage; the metaphyseal bone trabeculae are irregular. Osteoid seams (not seen here) may be present. The basic lesion is one of osteomalacia.

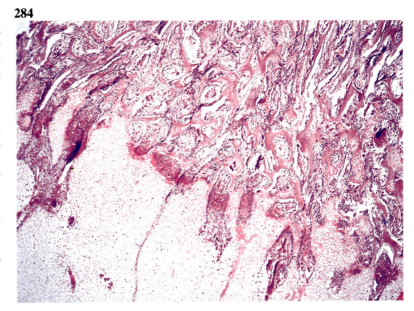

284

285 If bone mineralisation is sufficiently poor in young birds it may be possible to prepare undecalcified sections using normal equipment. Here, two such sections are compared. Figure **285A** is stained by the von Kossa method and demonstrates normal mineralisation in the metaphysis of an 8-day-old broiler. No mineral is detectable in the rachitic specimen from a 10-day-old broiler (**285B**). Von Kossa–van Gieson.

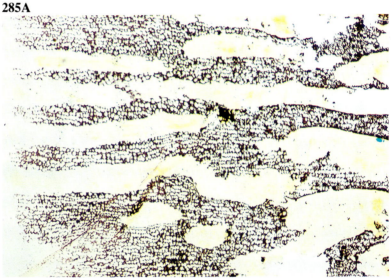

285A

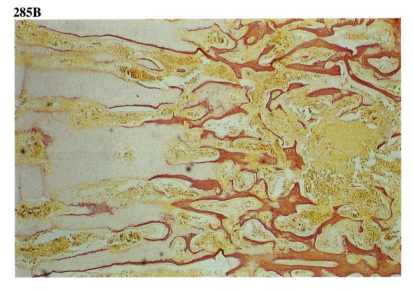

285B

286 In cases of phosphorus deficiency or calcium excess, the zone of hypertrophy in the physis is usually thickened but well vascularised by metaphyseal vessels. The chondrocyte columns remain regular. This example in a 3-week-old pheasant poult was attributed to an excess of calcium in the ration. Martius scarlet blue.

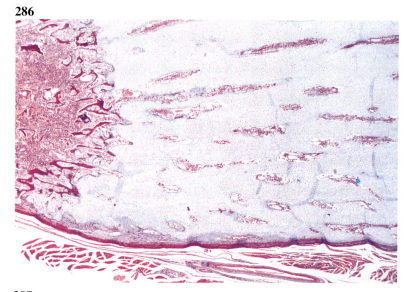

287 Enlargement of the parathyroid gland may be detectable in cases of calcium or vitamin D₃ deficiency. In this 2-week-old broiler, for example, the pale parathyroid (arrow) – though normally much smaller than the adjacent thyroid – is nearly as large. This feature is not usually seen in affected chicks or poults under 2 weeks of age.

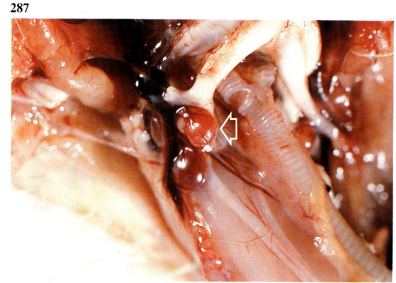

288 Cord-like arrangement of parenchymal cells and proliferation of stromal connective tissue, in an enlarged parathyroid gland from a severe case of hypocalcaemic rickets in a 3-week-old broiler. Acrylic resin, Lee's methylene blue-basic fushin.

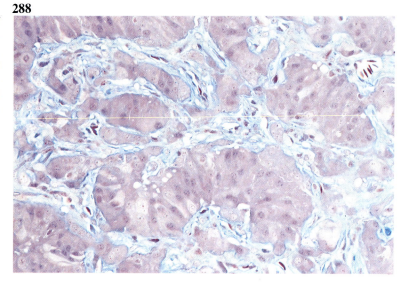

Osteopenia in adult laying fowl

Osteopenia is used here as a non-specific term to describe a decrease in the amount of bone tissue, such as can result from both osteomalacia and osteoporosis. While in osteomalacia there is defective mineralisation, in osteoporosis – though bone substance is lost – the matrix is mineralised normally.

Figures **289–291** illustrate an established case of calcium deficiency, such as might be expected to cause an osteomalacia. However, similar gross deformities may result from osteoporotic states, too. In fact, without histological examination it is difficult to decide whether lesions are osteomalacic or osteoporotic.

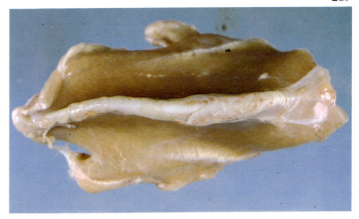

289 Calcium deficiency. Sternal deformity. The sternum and rib cage are frequently soft and distorted. Egg production drops and the shells are thin.

290 Calcium deficiency. Sigmoid flexure of the ventral part (arrows) of two ribs caused by pathological fractures.

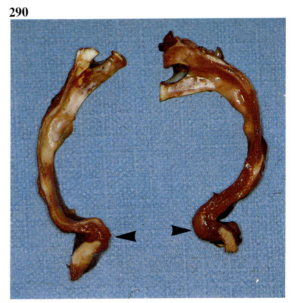

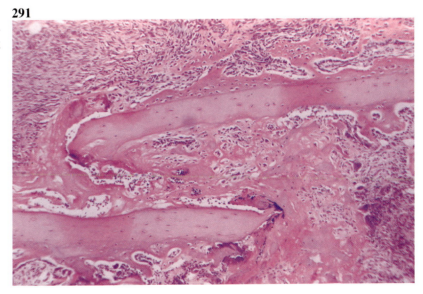

291 Calcium deficiency. The fractured rib seen in **290**. One cortex is shown.

292 Osteomalacia. Medullary bone with thick seams of osteoid in an adult layer.

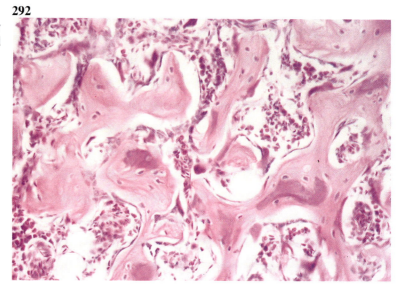

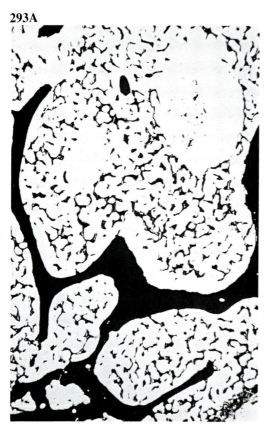

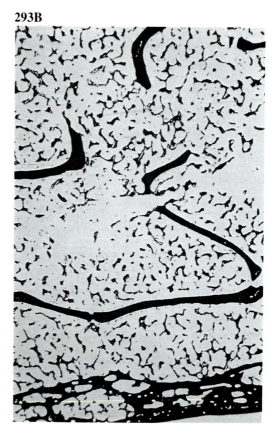

293 Osteoporosis. This lesion is encountered most frequently in caged laying fowl. Normal trabecular bone (**293A**) is compared to thin osteoporotic trabeculae (**293B**) in an adult layer. Bone cortices are usually thin and may contain resorption cavities. Undecalcified bone. Acrylic resin. Von Kossa.

294 Osteomalacia. Medullary bone (green) with red-staining osteoid in the same case as **292** on previous page. Undecalcified bone. Acrylic resin. Masson Goldner trichrome.

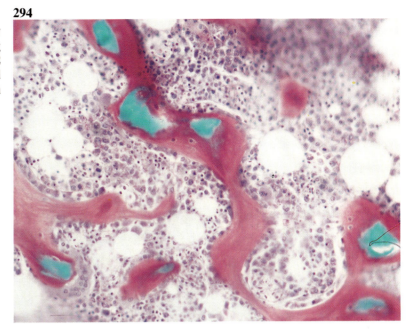

Fatty liver and kidney syndrome

295 The syndrome has been traditionally associated with broilers but has also been known to cause mortality in commercial layer chicks. Such chicks are seen here with ruffled feathers and suffering from depression, with some unable to rise from their hocks. Outbreaks of the disease have been largely prevented by the inclusion of additional biotin in rations.

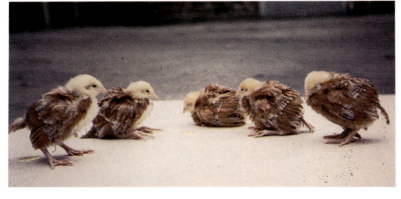

296 The subcutaneous fat is congested. This feature gave rise to the name 'pink disease'.

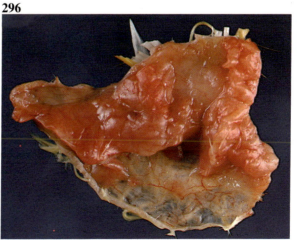

297 Livers are pale, often in a rather streaky fashion, and friable. It may be difficult to cut blocks of this tissue for fixation. Subcapsular haemorrhages may be present at necropsy, usually clustered near the posterior tips of the lobes.

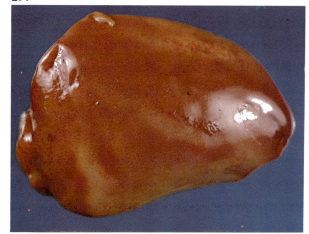

298 Most kidneys contain pale areas of tissue which contrast with the deep red colour of the normal organ. The kidney of this broiler was severely affected and had an even pallor. Note the outline of individual lobules within the renal divisions.

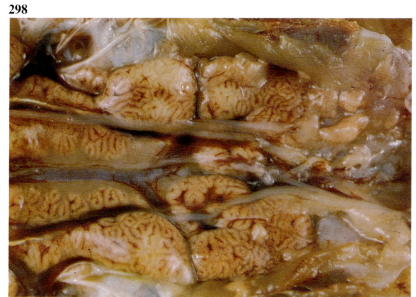

299 The pale appearance of the heart on the left, from an affected broiler, contrasts with the normal colour of the organ next to it, from an older bird.

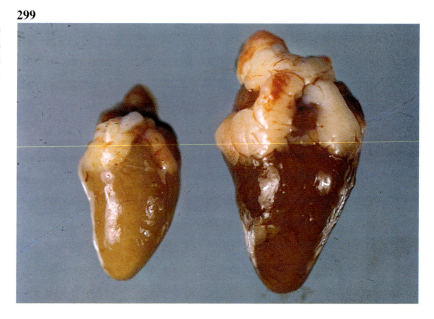

300 The small intestinal contents, especially those of the duodenum, may be very dark and possess a strong odour.

300

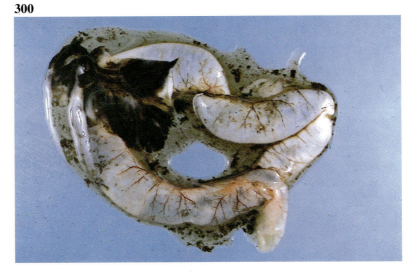

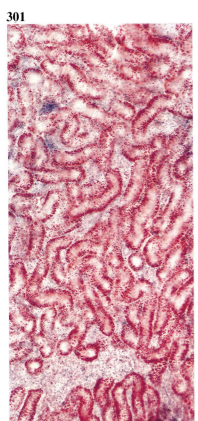

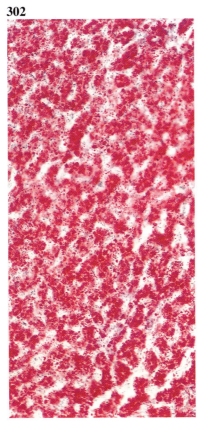

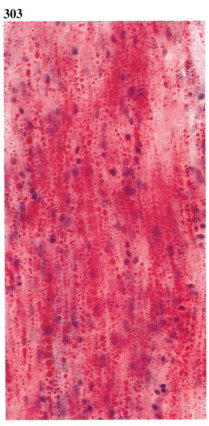

301 Histological confirmation of this disease requires demonstration of lipid in the kidney, liver and heart. Numerous fine lipid droplets are contained within the proximal convoluted tubular cells of this kidney. Oil red O.

302 Widespread distribution of fat in the hepatocytes of a broiler chick. Oil red O.

303 Fat droplets within the myocardium of a 14-day-old broiler. Oil red O.

Fatty liver haemorrhagic syndrome in laying fowl

304 A large blood clot surrounds the ruptured right lobe of the liver in an obese layer. Note the haemorrhages in the unruptured left lobe. The bird may survive several haemorrhagic episodes, particularly if escaping blood is confined within the lobes or as a subcapsular haematoma. The syndrome occurs in obese birds; both metabolic and environmental associations have been implicated.

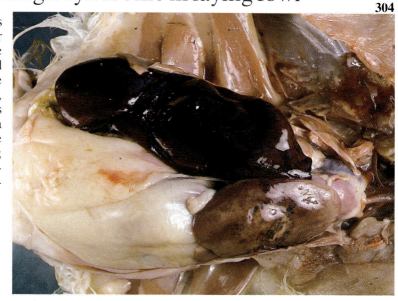

305 A blood clot emerging through a cut made in a subcapsular haematoma of the liver. Note the pale yellow colour of the hepatic tissue. Such tissue is usually extremely friable and it can be difficult to obtain suitable blocks for histology. It is often better to put large portions into fixative and trim after 24 hours.

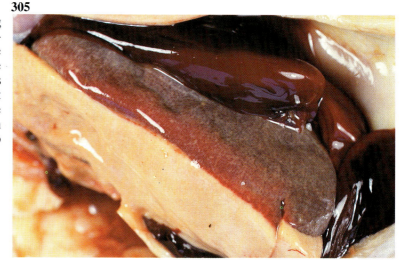

306 Death may occur in obese layers without haemorrhage taking place. The central liver lobe is a specimen from such a case. It is enlarged and very fatty, but not as severely affected as the ruptured specimen on the right. These lobes are compared with one on the left taken from a healthy bird in full lay. Note, too, how this lobe exhibits some streaking and pallor, which reflects the extent of lipid metabolism occurring in the normal liver of a layer.

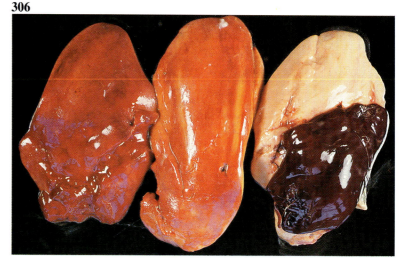

307 Excess fat in the ruptured liver of an obese layer. Sudan IV.

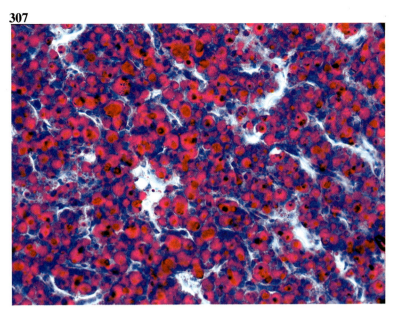

308 The presence of reticulin is demonstrated in the blood vessel walls but not in the surrounding hepatic parenchyma. The lesion has been described as a reticulolysis. Gordon and Sweet.

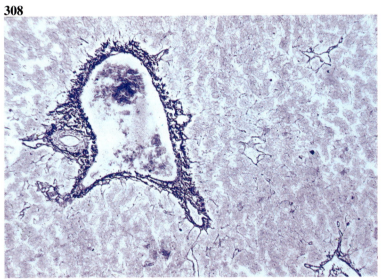

309 Reticulolysis is not always complete. This section demonstrates partial dissolution of the reticulin. Gordon and Sweet.

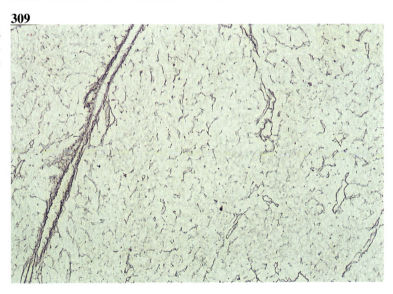

310 Reticulin network in a normal liver. Gordon and Sweet.

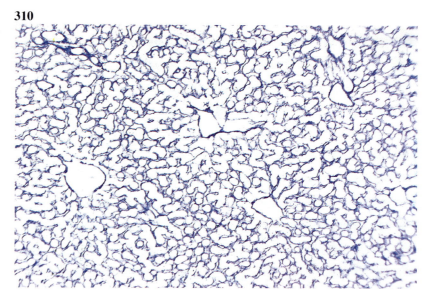

DISEASES OF UNCERTAIN OR UNKNOWN AETIOLOGY

Sudden death syndrome in broilers ('acute heart failure', 'flip-over')

311 This syndrome may cause death in broiler flocks from the end of the first week onwards, males being more frequently affected than females. Most carcases are found on their backs. Note the good condition of this carcase and the lack of any muscular congestion.

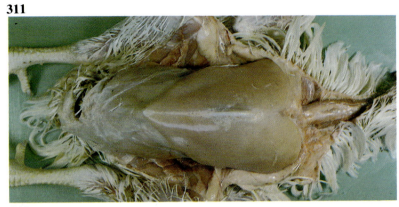

311

312 The digestive tract is full of food. There may be some pallor of the intestine, liver and kidneys. A congested lung (arrow) has been reflected from the rib cage in this 6-week-old broiler.

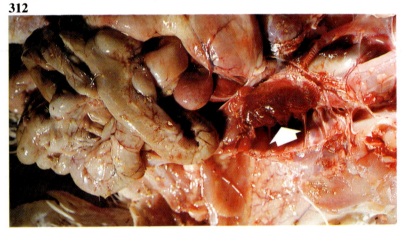

312

313 Bilateral pulmonary congestion and oedema is a common post-mortem finding and is usually sufficient to make the lungs turgid. These lungs were dissected from the broiler seen in figure **312**.

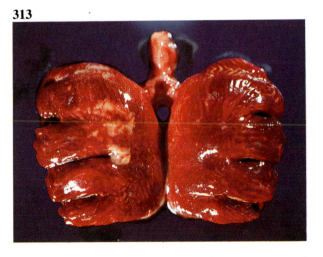

313

314 Pools of serosanguinous fluid often remain between the ribs after the lungs have been removed.

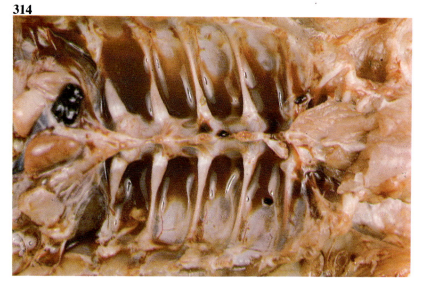

315 A section of lung confirms the intense congestion seen *post mortem*. In this specimen the airways are full of proteinaceous fluid (arrows), but the quantity and degree of eosinophilia vary considerably. There may be haemorrhages in the mucosa of the secondary bronchi.

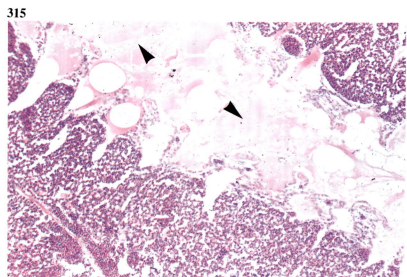

Sudden death syndrome in laying fowl

316 A common cause of sporadic death in both commercial and breeding birds that are in full lay. Protrusion of congested cloacal tissue through the vent is the only external feature.

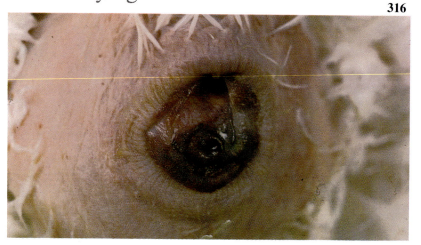

317 Intense congestion of the blood vessels on the surface of the ova and variable pulmonary congestion are frequently seen post-mortem features. A broken, shelled egg is sometimes found in the shell gland.

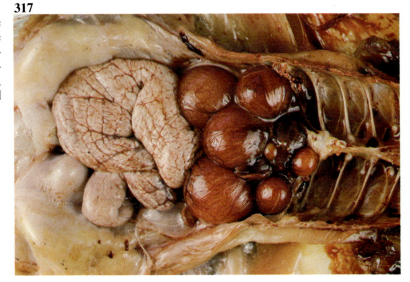

Cardiohepatic syndrome in turkeys

318 The syndrome typically occurs at 7–10 days of age, although it may be seen up to about 3 weeks. Poults are not usually observed ill but are found dead. Dilation of the right side of the heart, ascites, a pale and slightly 'brittle' liver, and generalised venous congestion are the main post-mortem features. The relationship of this syndrome to similar gross lesions in older turkeys is uncertain.

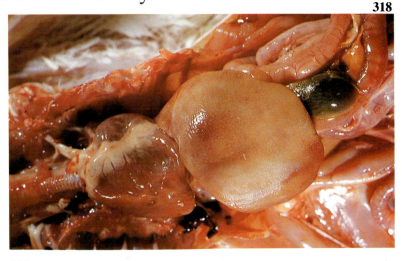

319 Dilated hearts from 3-week-old birds that probably survived from an earlier episode. Note the very thin-walled right ventricles from which blood has been expressed.

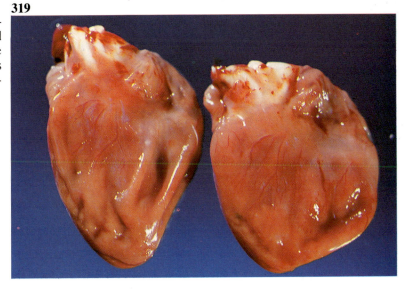

320 Liver sections reveal non-fatty vacuolation of hepatocytes and the presence of rounded PAS-positive cytoplasmic bodies. Early bile-duct proliferation may also be present. PAS-haematoxylin.

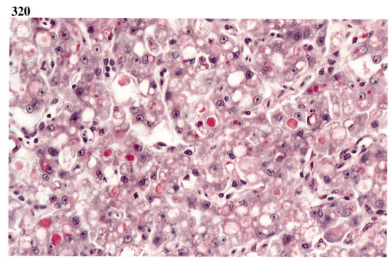

321 The rounded cytoplasmic bodies within degenerating hepatocytes also stain eosinophilically. Two such bodies (arrows) are seen near the centre of this photograph.

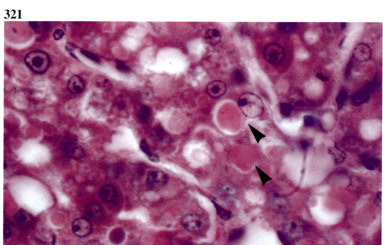

Right ventricular heart failure and ascites in broilers (broiler ascites)

322 A common disease occurring mainly in male broilers. Frequently seen as an incidental finding in many flocks but there may be outbreaks. There is severe ascites and a marked passive venous congestion throughout the carcase. Note the deep red colour of the musculature.

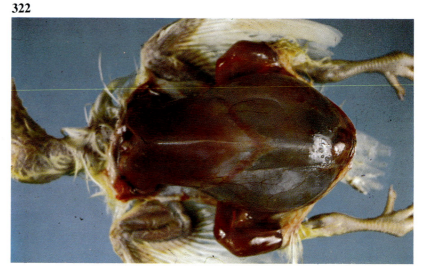

323 The ascitic fluid may be semi-clotted. The liver is small and has rounded borders. Dilation of the right side of the heart and intense passive congestion of the lungs and other viscera are the main post-mortem findings. Such changes are consistent with right-sided congestive heart failure and result from pulmonary hypertension.

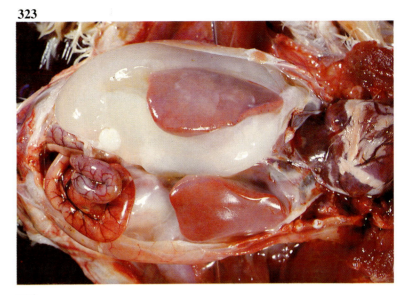

324 Comparison of cross-sections of fixed affected and unaffected hearts from 4-week-old broilers (the affected heart is shown above the unaffected heart). Note the right-sided dilation in the affected specimen.

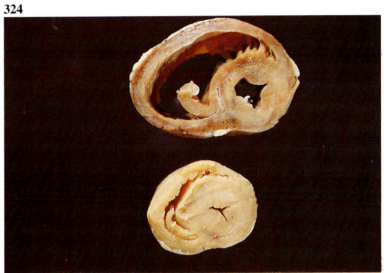

325 The apex of the heart has been reflected cranially to reveal a greatly distended posterior vena cava (arrow). Note the irregularity of the liver surface.

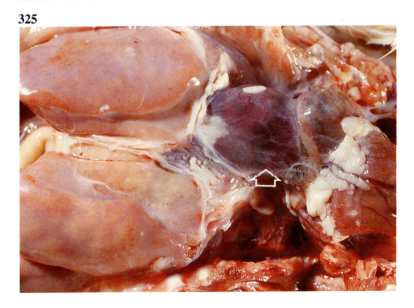

326 Lungs are congested and oedematous. An increase in the number of osseous foci is sometimes apparent and here in an experimental bird there are exceptional numbers. Masson's trichrome.

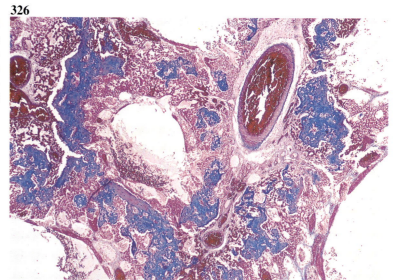

327 Liver from a chronically affected broiler with pallor and rounding of borders.

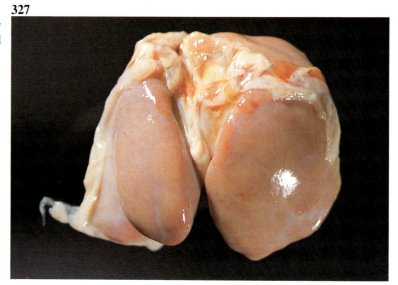

328 Low-power view of a chronic liver lesion. A fibrinous deposit is present over the capsule. Other features include dilation of the intrahepatic branches of the hepatic vein and patchy condensation of parenchymal connective tissue. Martius scarlet blue.

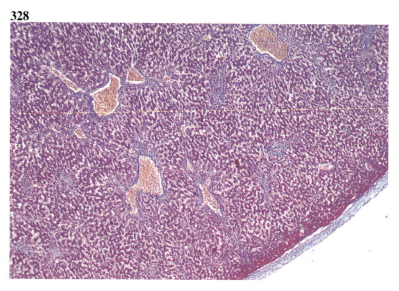

329 Dead birds are also found in affected flocks with hepatic lesions that represent an earlier stage of the disease. Grossly, such livers are swollen and discoloured, and often have a mottled or dimpled surface. In this specimen dimpling is not present but a fine reticular pattern of pale bands of tissue can be seen through the capsule. There may be little or no ascites at this stage.

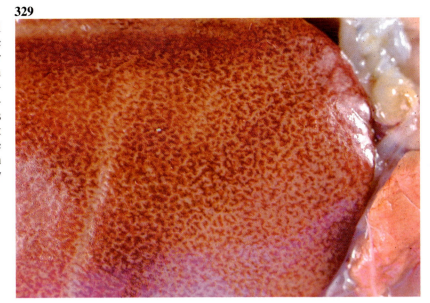

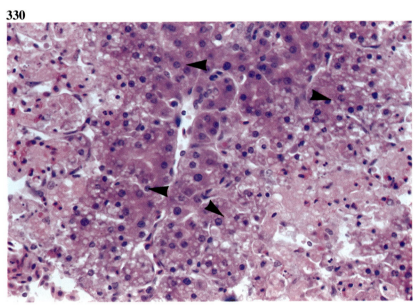

330 Sections from a liver such as that in **329** reveal, initially, a marked hepatocytic fatty change that mainly affects periacinar tissue. This is quickly succeeded by coagulative necrosis of the affected zones. Here, a central band of surviving hepatocytes is flanked by degenerating cells on either side, vacuolation (fatty) being apparent at the junctions (arrows) of the viable and degenerating hepatocytes. These changes are probably caused by an anoxia resulting from progressive heart failure. Haemorrhagic replacement and heterophilic infiltration are variable features of such lesions.

Round heart disease

331 This disease is now uncommon, but at one time it was seen as a cause of sudden death during winter months in fowls maintained on deep litter. The enlarged heart usually has a blunted apex in which there may be a central depression. Compare with the normal heart, left.

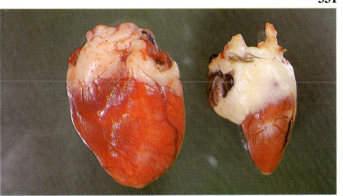

332 Degenerative fatty changes in swollen heart muscle fibres cut in cross-section. Note also the nuclear degeneration.

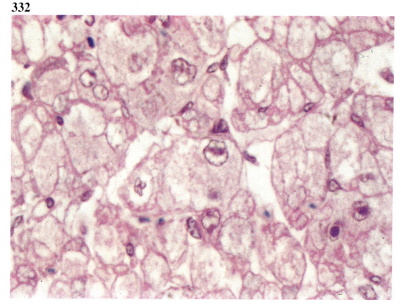

Focal hepatic lipidosis

333 Seen usually as an incidental post-mortem finding in adult laying fowl, the lesion requires differentiation from focal necrosis which, grossly, it may resemble. Discrete pale foci tend to be scattered throughout the liver and vary greatly in number and size. Histologically, such lesions are composed of rounded clumps of hepatocytes that have undergone fatty change and which are clearly demarcated from the surrounding parenchyma.

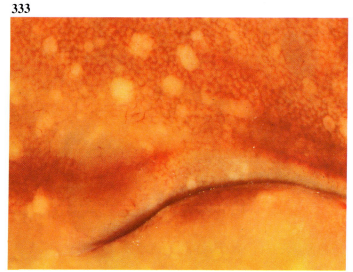

Dermatitis in broilers

334 This form of dermatitis has appeared sporadically in Britain. Clinical signs are not usually reported, nor are lesions apparent until after slaughter, when the plucking of the carcases often reveals well-defined areas of thickened and discoloured skin on the thighs, which may extend on to the back.

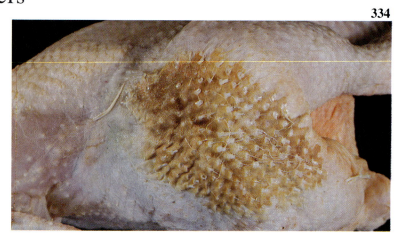

335A

335B

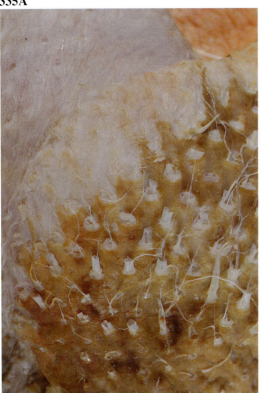

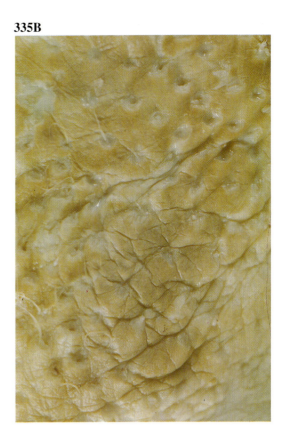

335 The surface of the lesion is slightly raised above the level of the surrounding normal skin and is usually yellow or brown in colour. Specimen **335A** is a closer view of the lesion seen in **334**. The brown material is a fine scab which is on the point of separating; more often the surface has a yellowish discoloration (**335B**) and a scab is not distinguishable grossly.

336 Flattened plaques of purulent material frequently lie in the subcutaneous tissue. When these are peeled away fine haemorrhages may be observed on the surface of the limb muscles.

336

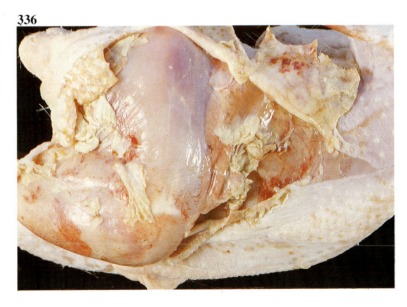

337 Histologically, early lesions consist of an inflammatory oedema of the dermis and epidermal necrosis. Small clumps of Gram-negative bacteria (not present here) are often visible deep in the inflammatory reaction. Cultural examination may yield growths of *Escherichia coli* and, occasionally, *Pasteurella multocida*; the significance of these bacteria and their mode of entry are uncertain. Tracts of purulent debris appear in the subcutaneous fat.

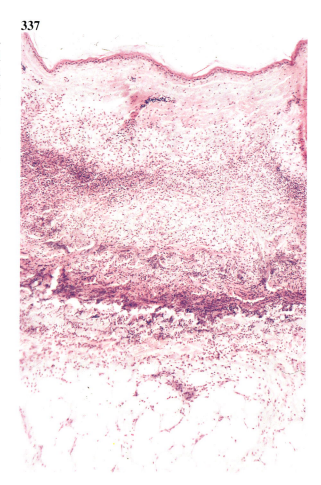

337

Cholangiohepatitis in broilers

338

338 Affected birds are usually detected at slaughter and in most cases there is no flock history of illness or rise in mortality. Liver enlargement is obvious and there may be jaundice of the carcase. The presence of jaundiced ascitic fluid is variable.

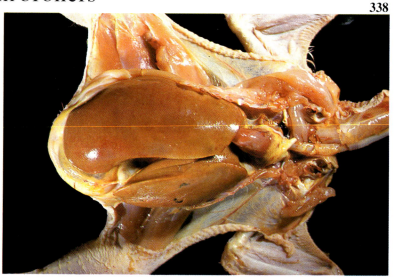

339 The enlarged livers are very firm on palpation. In some, a regular pattern of pale lesions is visible beneath the capsule. This pattern is less reticular than that seen in right ventricular heart failure of broilers (*see* **329**).

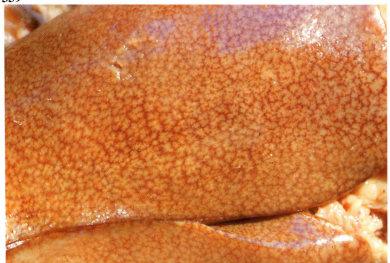

340 Cholecystitis and cholangitis of the extrahepatic bile ducts are frequently observed. When opened, the enlarged gall bladder and bile ducts of this specimen contained yellow inspissated material. *Clostridium perfringens* is often isolated from the gall bladder contents and the liver. Occasionally, concurrent lesions of inclusion body hepatitis have been observed in early cases. A segment of duodenum has been left attached to the extrahepatic ducts.

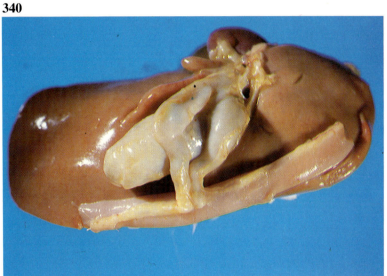

341 A complex lesion is seen histologically. The principal change is one of bile-duct proliferation and accompanying fibrosis (seen low power as the pale tissue in this section). Hepatocytic cords are still apparent but may all but disappear. The more dense eosinophilic areas in the lower part of the photograph consist of masses of immature granulocytes.

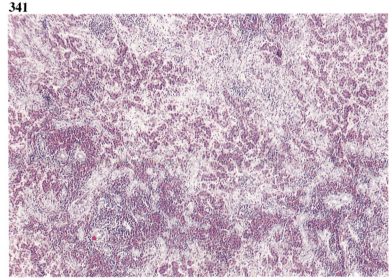

342 Pale-staining proliferating bile ducts are surrounded by a delicate network of connective tissue. A few mauve-coloured hepatocytes are still identifiable in the centre of the picture. Note the scattered clumps of granulocytes. These lesions start periportally and spread to form bridges with adjoining triads. Intrahepatic cholangitis is variable but there is usually some evidence of biliary stasis and inflammation. The immature appearance of the granulocytes and the presence of mitoses amongst this population suggest that at least part of the infiltration is caused by extramedullary granulopoiesis. Lymphocytic infiltration may also take place. Acrylic resin. Trichrome.

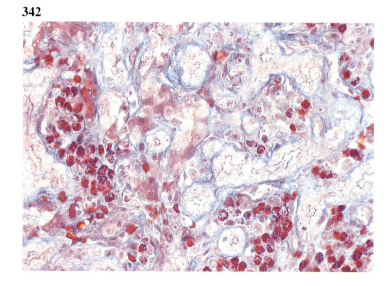

342

Dyschondroplasia

343 Seen in both broilers and turkey growers. It is more common in male birds. This physeal cartilage abnormality may be present at the ends of all the long bones in the leg and has been reported in the humerus. The tibiotarsus is most frequently affected, and in this 6-week-old broiler the upper part of the bone is severely deformed.

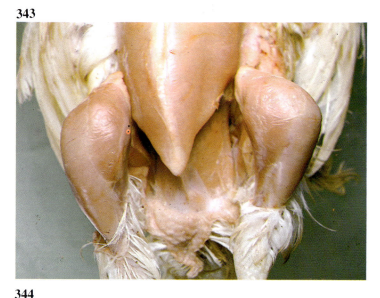

343

344 The top bone is a tibiotarsus removed from the broiler in **343**, which has been split to show the large posteriorly bent head containing a plug of abnormal physeal cartilage (arrows). Pathological fractures are present on both the anterior and the posterior aspects. The bone below is normal.

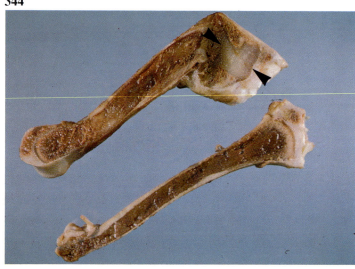

344

345 The head of this tibiotarsus is also bent posteriorly. A large mass of abnormal cartilage extends from the physis into the metaphysis.

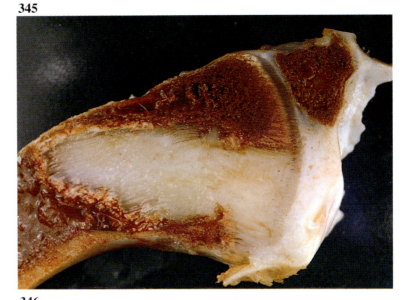

346 The lesion has been partially resolved in this bone, but a substantial quantity of abnormal cartilage remains.

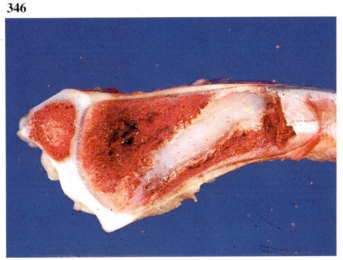

347 These specimens were obtained from an 8-week-old broiler in a flock where birds were reported with gait abnormalities. The large proximal lesions in the tibiotarsus and tarsometatarsus were bilateral. Note the scabs just below the posterior aspect of the hock joint (centre), probably resulting from increased contact with litter. Many broilers may be affected by dyschondroplasia but do not develop leg deformity or gait abnormalities unless the lesions are large.

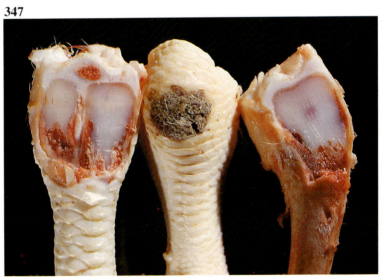

348 Low-power view of a shallow dyschondroplastic lesion in the proximal tarsometatarsus of a broiler. Martius scarlet blue.

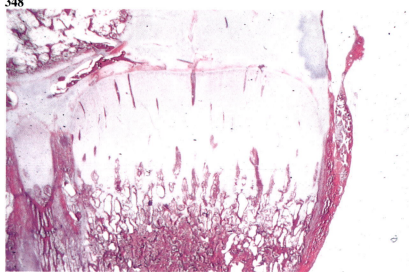

349 An area of abnormal cartilage in the metaphysis. The metaphyseal blood vessels are numerous but those near the periphery of the cartilage appear empty (arrows) and hardly invade the cartilage. Martius scarlet blue.

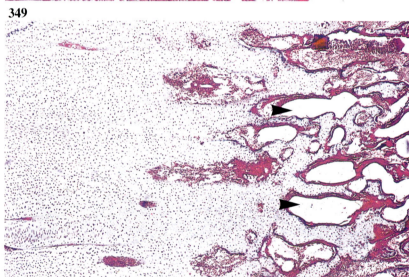

350 The lack of blood supply to the pre-hypertrophied cartilage leads to necrosis of the distal cells. Necrotic cartilage cells contain eosinophilic nuclei in this field.

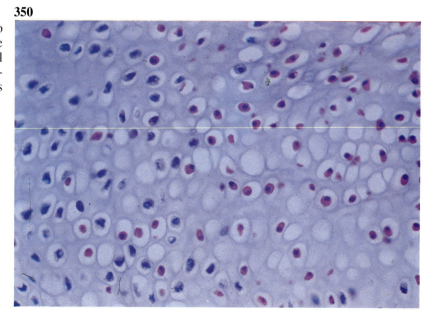

Valgus leg deformity in broilers ('twisted leg')

351 Valgus deformity is seen from about 2 weeks of age onwards, and occurs more often in males than in females. One leg or both may be affected, the deformity causing the leg to bend outwards at the hock joint. The bilaterally affected specimen is shown from the posterior aspect.

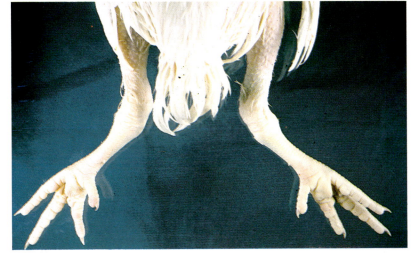

351B

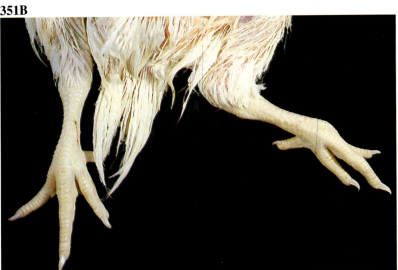

352

352 Removal of the musculature shows that in most cases the deformity results from a lateral tilting (rather than twisting) of the distal tibiotarsal condyles. Anterior aspect.

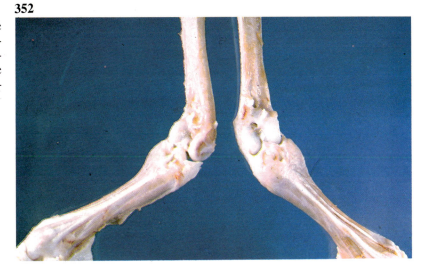

353 Progressively severe angular deformity affecting three legs from left to right. As the angulation becomes more extreme the gastrocnemius tendon slips from its normal location and usually comes to lie laterally over the bone. Anterior aspect.

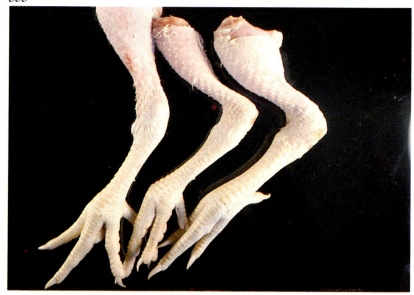

354 The lateral deviation of the distal tibiotarsal condyles may be sufficiently severe for the condyles to become separated from the shaft of the bone. In this broiler the shaft has come to lie underneath the skin just above the hock joint.

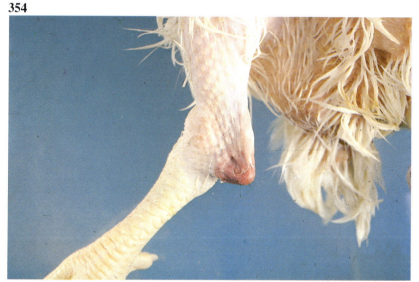

355 A dissected hock joint of a broiler shows the condyles at right angles to the shaft of the bone. Dyschondroplasia may be found in the distal tibiotarsus of some severely deformed cases.

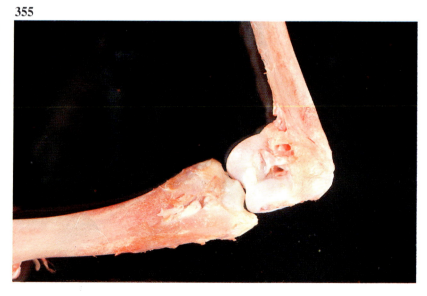

Twisted leg in turkeys

356 The lower third of the bottom tibiotarsus has rotated laterally. This process produces a similar overall effect to valgus deformity of the legs in broilers ('twisted leg'), but it is usually restricted to one leg and is a true rotation of the shaft. It is occasionally seen in broilers.

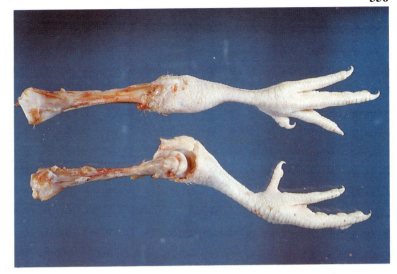

357 The limb rotation sometimes exceeds 90°. In this 4-week-old turkey it approached 180°. The posterior aspect of the affected leg on the left is therefore seen alongside the anterior view of the opposite limb.

357

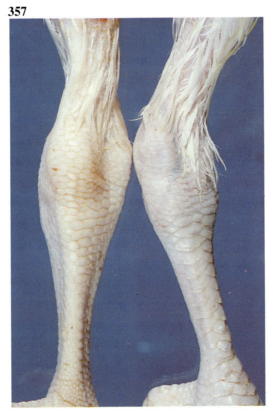

Renal failure (visceral gout)

Renal failure is a common cause of death in fowls of different types and ages. It is also seen in the turkey. Apart from recognised causes of renal disease such as nephritis induced by infectious bronchitis virus, water deprivation, and excessive intake of protein and calcium, the aetiology of many of the nephritides and nephroses is uncertain. Visceral gout, i.e. the deposition of urates on the surfaces of the viscera and in the joints, should not be regarded as a single entity, but rather as an end stage of, possibly, many different renal diseases. Generally, kidney disease is more prevalent in adult laying fowl.

The post-mortem appearance of avian kidneys is often deceptive. It is usually difficult to say from any gross abnormalities that may be present whether they represent inflammatory or non-inflammatory states. Unless the cause of such changes is clear (e.g. when uroliths are present), it is inadvisable either to apply such terms as 'nephritis' or 'nephrosis' without the support of a histological examination, or to assume that the changes represent an example of a primary renal disease. One of the commonest post-mortem findings, for example, is the presence of pale swollen kidneys in which excess urates can be detected in the subcapsular tissue. Attention is drawn elsewhere (**51**, **59**) to examples of non-specific changes of this type that may accompany some bacterial infections and toxaemias. They may be the most striking of post-mortem findings, which can therefore make it a little surprising histologically if, from what was a grossly abnormal organ, all that is found with conventional light microscopy is a restricted tubular dilation. In spite of the fact that there may be a poor correlation between the gross and microscopic appearances in these cases, it is still necessary to perform such examinations in order to attempt further interpretation. It is clear that changes frequently occur in the kidneys of birds that are ill from a number of different causes. It is possible that variations in the amount of blood and waste products contained within them may produce subtle alterations in the spatial relationships of tubules and vessels, which in turn affect the macroscopic appearance.

Two lesions of known cause (**375**, **376**) are included in this section for comparative purposes.

358 Baby chick nephropathy. Lesions occur during the first week of life and may cause heavy mortality, with some birds dying shortly after hatching. The kidneys are swollen and pale, and urates are usually deposited on the viscera and in the joints. Five-day-old broiler.

358

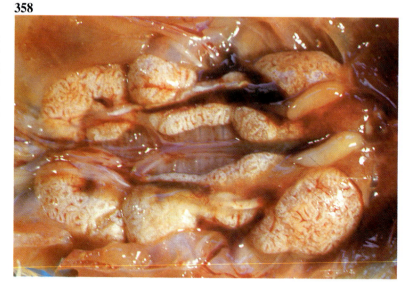

359 Baby chick nephropathy. Urate deposits in the toe joints of this broiler chick can be seen through the skin.

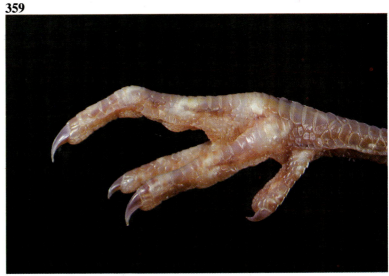

360 Baby chick nephropathy. Histologically, lesions tend to be of two types. In one form (**360A**), there is dilation of ureteral branches and of some medullary tract collecting ducts. Inflammation is usually mild or absent. This kidney is compared with normal tissue (**360B**); note here the basophilic tissue at the periphery of the lobules, which is a normal feature of the young bird, caused by the presence of undifferentiated embryonic nephrons.

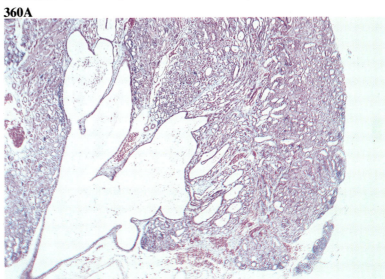

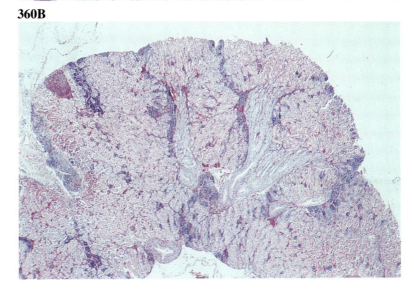

361 Baby chick nephropathy. The second type of lesion seen in this nephropathy is an interstitial nephritis characterised by the presence of multifocal tubular necroses in the cortex, cellular casts and urate deposits. It is not known what relationship, if any, exists between the lesions in this form and those illustrated in **360**.

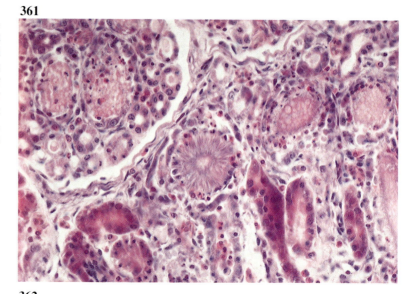

362 Urolithiasis. This lesion is more prevalent in laying fowl, affected birds usually remaining in lay until shortly before death. One or both kidneys show signs of atrophy, and the carcases are congested. The ureters are greatly distended (arrows) with mucus and uroliths.

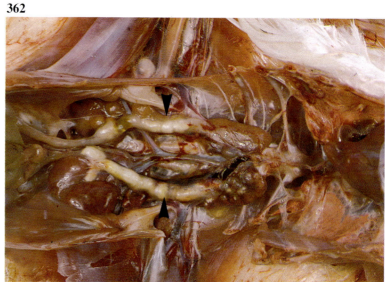

363 Urolithiasis. This adult broiler breeder hen died in good bodily condition. One kidney has almost completely atrophied, and compensatory hypertrophy has taken place in the divisions of the opposite organ, which is drained by a large distended ureter (arrows). Urates are present on the surface of the epicardium. In some birds, a single hypertrophied division is all that may remain at the time of death.

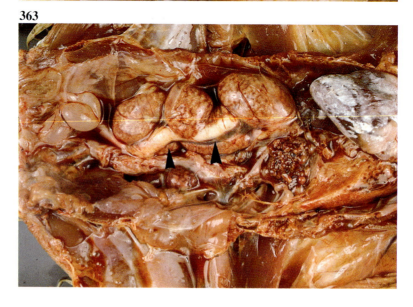

364 Urolithiasis. A greatly distended ureter on the left almost obscures the atrophic kidney on that side, and compensatory hypertrophy has taken place on the right. These kidneys were dissected from an adult commercial layer.

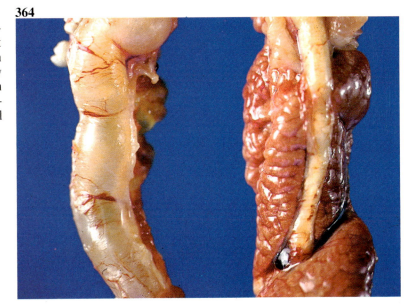

365 Urolithiasis. A ureter has been opened immediately distal to a hypertrophied anterior division to reveal a large urolith (arrow, **365A**). Two small uroliths (**365B**) can be seen emerging through the ureteral openings in the cloaca of another bird.

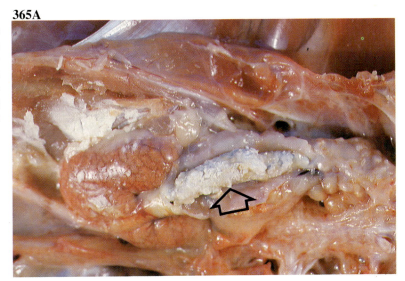

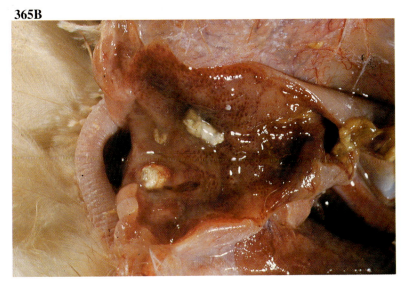

366 Urolithiasis. Dilated collecting tubules in a medullary tract of an adult laying fowl. Masses of inflammatory cells are present within the tubules, and there is usually an interstitial nephritis. This lesion is commonly seen but is of doubtful specificity.

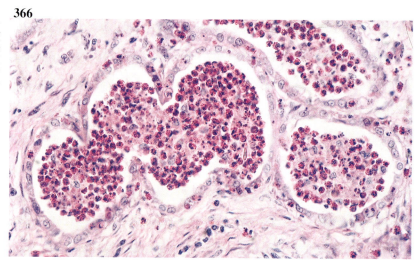

367 Urolithiasis. A focal area of necrosis within the cortex, probably resulting from coalescing degenerate proximal convoluted tubules. Note the dilation of the surrounding tubules and the flattening of their epithelium. Focal lesions of this type are often seen in cases of interstitial nephritis due to other causes.

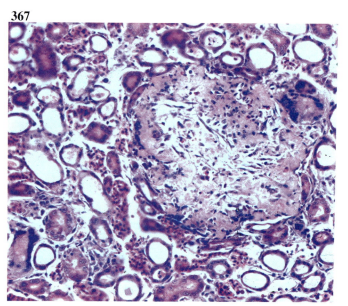

368 Visceral gout. Urates present on the surface of the liver, abdominal fat and sternum, the reflective quality of these deposits helping to distinguish them from inflammatory exudates.

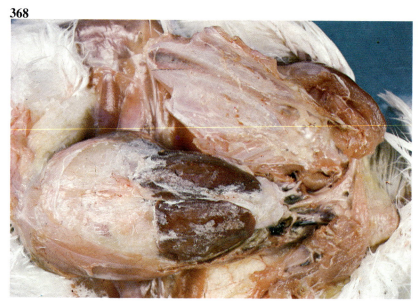

369 Visceral gout. Urates contained within a hock joint.

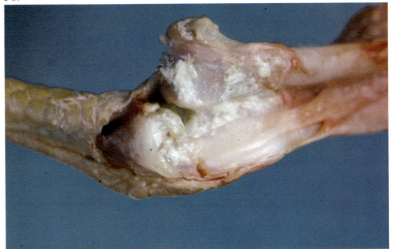

370 Visceral gout. Tophus formation may occur terminally in the kidney and other tissues such as the liver and spleen. Such a lesion is represented here as the presence of multiple pale foci over the cut surface of a liver lobe from a 20-week-old laying fowl.

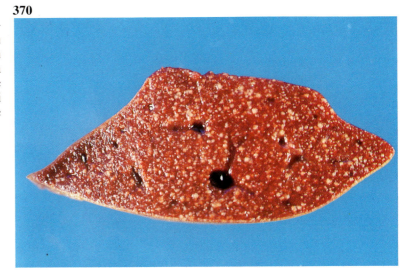

371 Visceral gout. Tophus formation in a section of liver from a similar specimen to that shown in **370**. The lesion consists of a necrotic subcapsular focus. Urates have dissolved out of the tissue during processing but the crystalline pattern of their deposition is still visible.

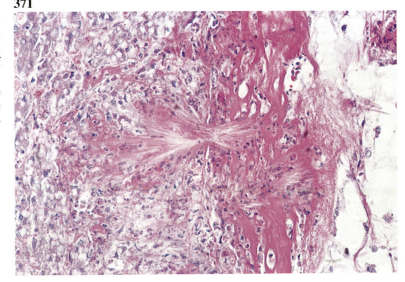

372 Visceral gout. Tophus formation within the cortical tissue of a kidney (tissue fixed in absolute alcohol and stained by the Gomori methenamine silver method).

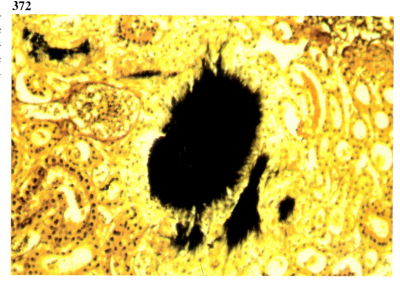

372

373 Glomerulopathy of unknown cause in an adult laying fowl. Mesangial proliferation is evident in the tuft in **373A**, while that in **373B** is becoming obsolescent and is accompanied by a thickening of Bowman's capsule and periglomerular fibrosis. Lesions of this type are encountered occasionally but do not appear to be of economic significance. PAS-haematoxylin. Acrylic resin.

373A

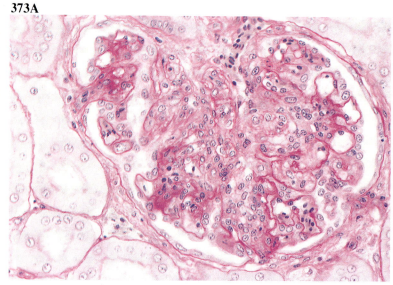

373B

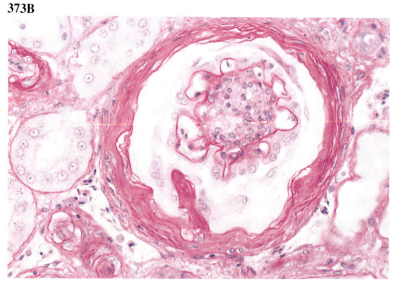

374 Visceral gout. Multiple splenic tophi have stimulated an early giant-cell response at their periphery. Adult laying fowl.

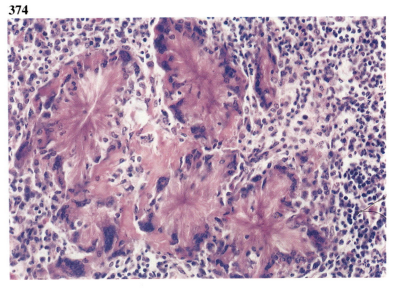

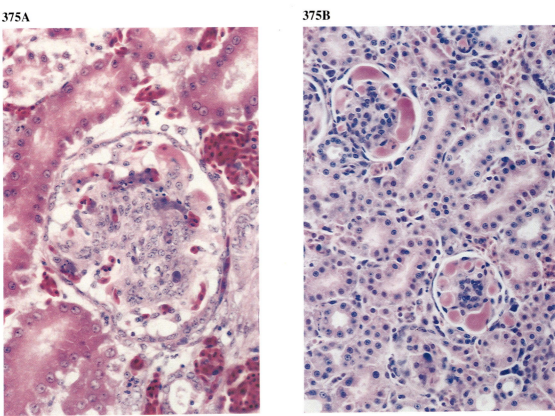

375 Glomeruli containing intra-capillary fibrinous thrombi. The lesion is encountered in some bacterial septicaemias, more often in young birds. The tissue in **375A** is from a case of colisepticaemia in a 15-week-old turkey. Basophilically staining bacteria are also present in the capillaries of the tuft. These features are compared with a kidney (**375B**) from a case of chlamydiosis in a psittacine, in which similar glomerular lesions are present.

376 Ethylene glycol toxicity may cause renal oxalosis. Birefringence of tubular deposits of oxalates is seen in a section of kidney from an affected peafowl. The crystals tend to be fan-shaped.

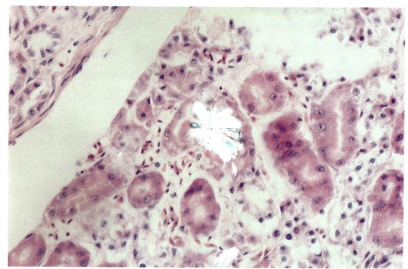

377 Articular gout. Periarticular deposits of urates in two feet (the normal foot is on the right for comparison). The aetiology is distinct from that of visceral gout.

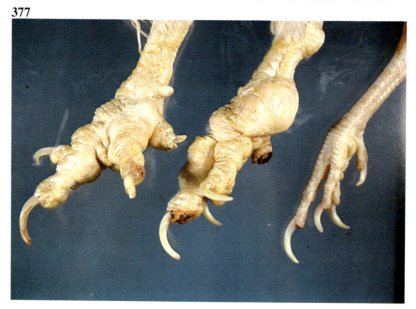

Infectious stunting syndrome in the fowl

378 Though occurring more frequently in broilers, this disease is also seen in commercial layer replacements. The clinical signs and post-mortem findings vary between countries. In Britain it has been more noticeable clinically during the second week of life; both the broilers shown are 23 days of age. Note the retention of chick down on the small bird and also the abdominal protrusion. Abnormalities of the primary wing feathers may result in a 'helicopter' appearance.

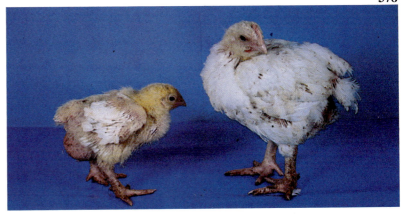

379 Gross lesions vary in different outbreaks. One of the features of the disease in Britain has been the appearance of pancreatic lesions in some of the affected birds at about 2 weeks of age. A pale fibrosed pancreas in a stunted 5-week-old is compared with the normal gland in a 3-week-old specimen from the same farm (the normal gland is shown above the fibrosed pancreas). Pancreatic tissue at the closed end of the duodenal loop is usually affected first. This lesion arises from inflammation and obstruction of the pancreatic ducts.

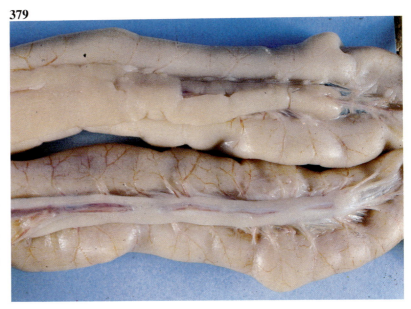

380 Early stages of degeneration, atrophy and fibrosis are taking place in the exocrine tissue of this pancreas. There is a marked vacuolation of the acinar cells, and only a few of these contain zymogen granules. Acrylic resin.

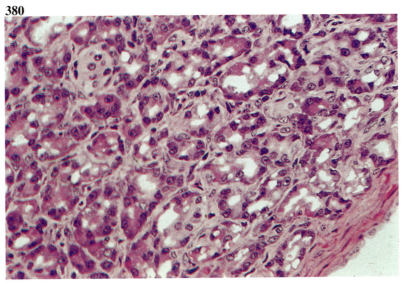

381 A scanning view (**381A**) of a severely affected pancreatic lobe reveals extensive atrophy of exocrine tissue and fibrous replacement. Note the darker-staining rounded foci which are seen (**381B**) to consist of acini that still have a normal zymogen content and which are situated around islets of Langerhans. This islet-sparing effect on contiguous exocrine tissue may be prominent.

381A

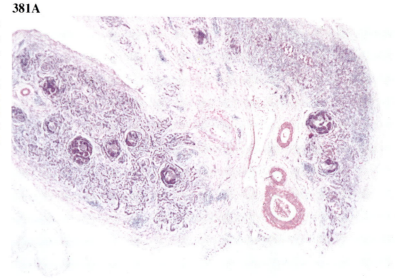

381B

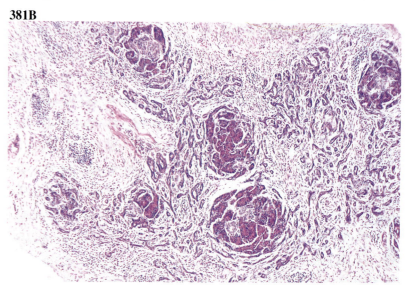

382 Side view of the distended abdomen in a 2-week-old broiler.

382

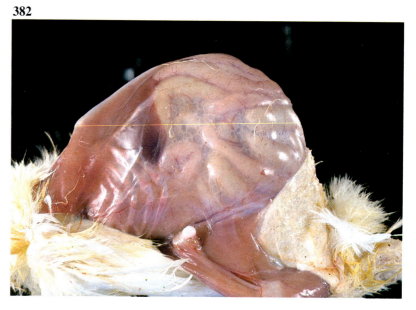

383 The intestines are pale and dilated, this dilation giving rise to the abdominal distension. Undigested food is present in the lower bowel. The pale pancreas (arrow) can be seen in the duodenal loop.

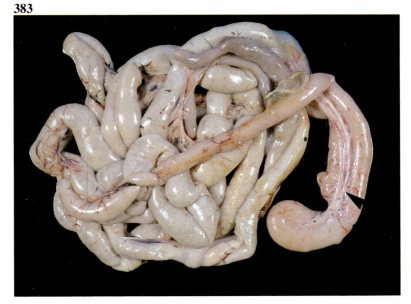

384 Some sections of the small intestine in affected chicks reveal cystic dilation of the crypts of Lieberkühn. The lesions are most noticeable under 10 days of age. An oblique section gives a false impression of a thickened mucosa in this specimen.

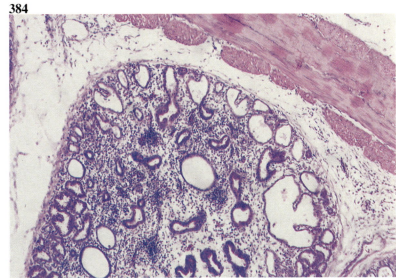

385 Poorly digested food in the lower small intestine and caeca of a broiler.

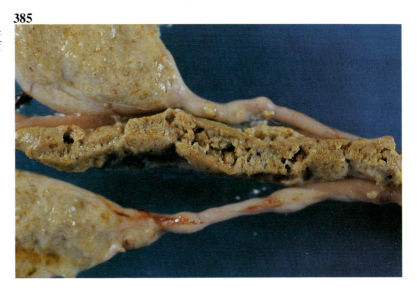

386 Osteodystrophic changes may affect the skeleton. Note the swollen rib heads from a stunted broiler on the left compared to a normal specimen (*see* **282**).

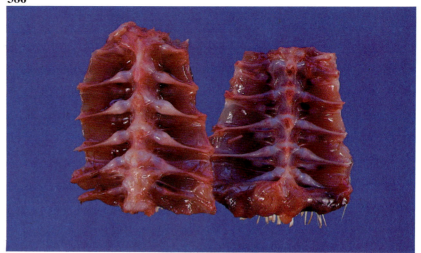

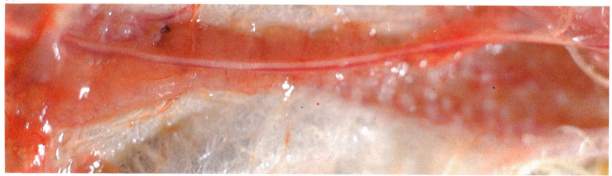

387 Atrophy of the thymus in a 3-week-old broiler. As viewed, the vagal nerve lies over small reddened portions of the gland.

Acute pectoral myopathy in broiler breeders

388 A sporadically occurring lesion that is more often encountered during rearing. Affected birds are not usually seen ill. Gelatinous fluid is frequently present in the subcutaneous tissue overlying the breast and also separates muscle fibre groups within the *Musculus pectoralis*, particularly in the deeper parts of this muscle. Pools of this fluid may collect between the *M. pectoralis* and the *M. supracoracoideus*.

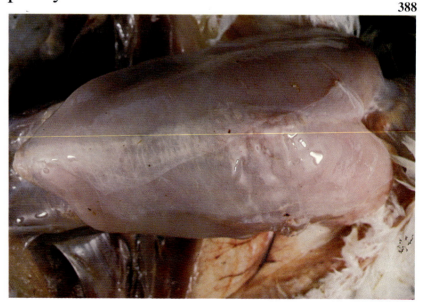

389 Severe myodegeneration in a *M. pectoralis*. Masson's trichrome.

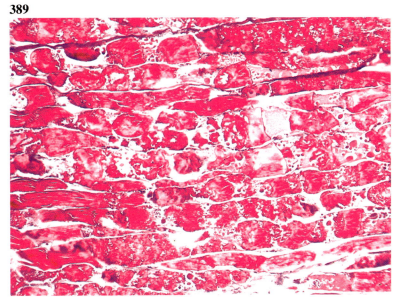

390 Contraction of necrotic segments of cytoplasm in three fibres of the *M. pectoralis*. Note the pale blue staining fluid filling the emptied portions of the endomysial tubes. Masson's trichrome.

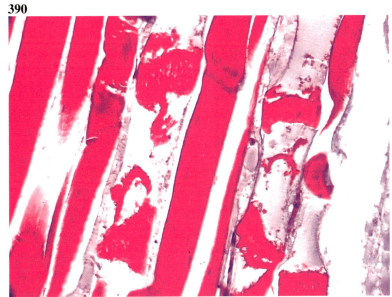

MISCELLANEOUS DISEASES

Spondylolisthesis (kinky back)

391 Clinical cases are usually seen in broilers between 3 and 6 weeks of age. Birds squat back on their hocks and cannot stand. One or both feet are often slightly raised from the surface on which they are placed.

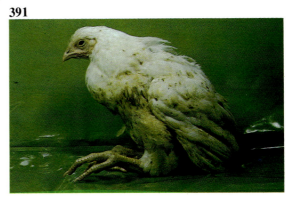

392 The disease is caused by a ventral rotation of the cranial end of the fourth thoracic vertebra (T4, formerly described as T6). This results in a dorsal displacement of the caudal end of T4, which may then compress the spinal cord (arrow) – particularly if the interarticular facets fail between T4 and T5.

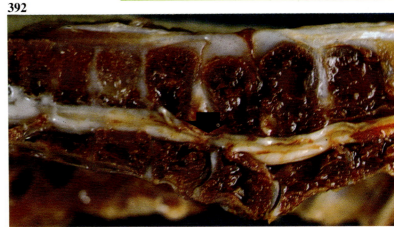

393 Spinal cord with compressed zone (arrow).

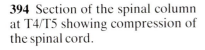

394 Section of the spinal column at T4/T5 showing compression of the spinal cord.

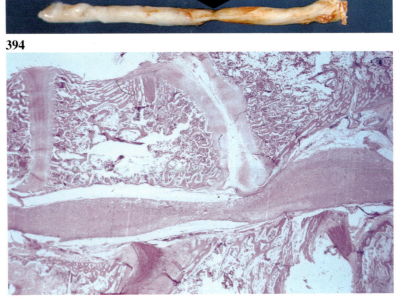

395 Spondylitis often affects the caudal thoracic vertebrae in broilers and is introduced here because of the similarity of the clinical signs to those of kinky back. The compression of the cord is clearly seen but note that it is the swelling of the infected focus that has caused the compression, not vertebral rotation. Seven-week-old broiler. A variety of organisms may be associated with such lesions including streptococci, staphylococci and some fungi.

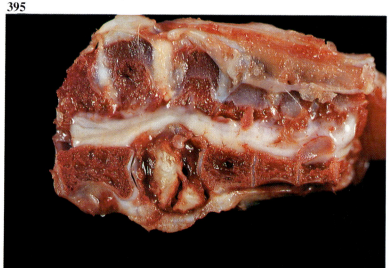

Ruptured gastrocnemius tendon

396 Spontaneous rupture of the tendon may occur sporadically, usually in heavy fowl such as capons and broiler breeders, although it is occasionally seen as an outbreak. The lesion may be unilateral or bilateral. Viral arthritis should be suspected if the rupture has been preceded by a chronic tendinitis and tenosynovitis (*see* **167**).

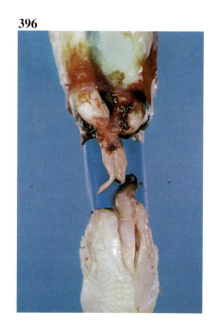

Deep pectoral myopathy

397 Occurs in turkeys and broiler breeders. The lesion is usually observed at meat inspection, and may affect either one or both of the deep pectoral muscles (*Musculus supracoracoideus*). This turkey breeder carcase has dished pectoral musculature on the right of the photograph. A black line has been drawn over the breast to distinguish the two sides.

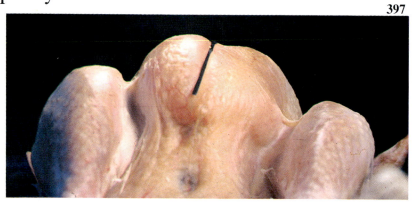

398 The *M. supracoracoideus* is contained in an osteofascial compartment. Abnormal exercise for birds of this type, such as the undue flapping of wings, may in some individuals lead to a swelling of the muscle and occlusion of its blood supply. Necrosis results. The fascia of the muscle of this 33-week-old broiler breeder has been cut anteriorly to show the bulging affected tissue (arrows) of the acute lesion. The early lesion may be accompanied by the production of gelatinous fluid.

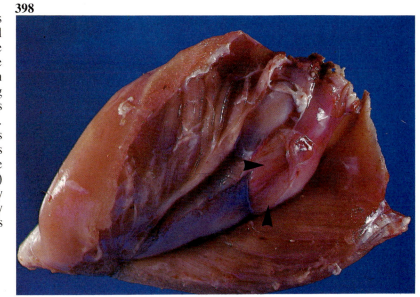

399 The bottom muscle is an affected *M. supracoracoideus* that is undergoing atrophy. Most of the necrotic tissue lies centrally. The small size of this muscle contrasts with a normal dissected specimen above. The medio-ventral aspect is shown.

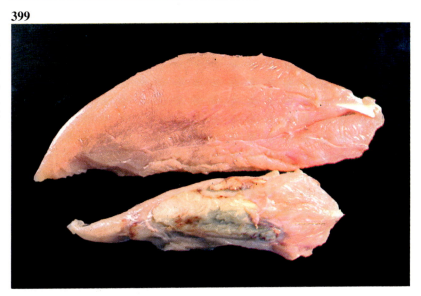

400 The necrotic tissue is often an unusual apple-green colour and tends to be dry and crumbly. Broiler breeder, 30 weeks of age.

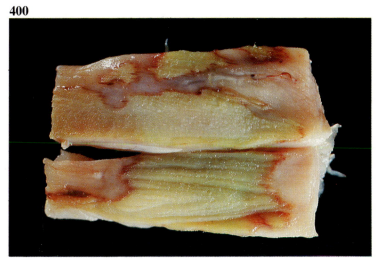

401 Cooked lesion. The green colour is retained.

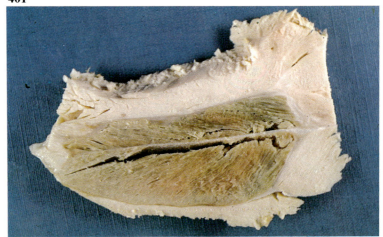

402 Fragments of necrotic *M. supracoracoideus* (arrows) adhering to the sternum of a turkey breeder.

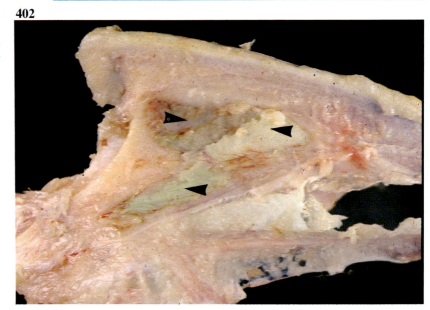

403 Junctions of normal and affected *M. supracoracoideus*. The necrotic tissue below is staining more palely with eosin than the viable muscle above.

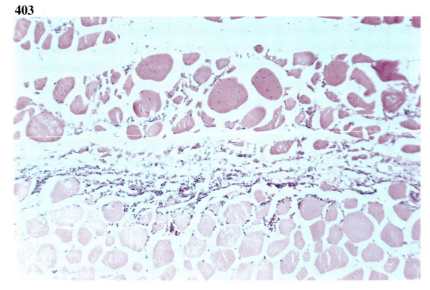

404 Muscle fibres within an affected *M. supracoracoideus*, exhibiting discoid necrosis.

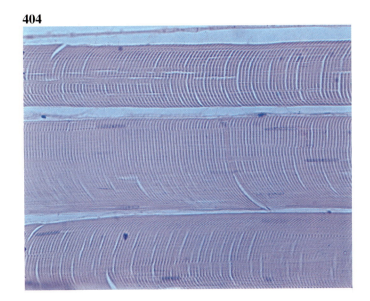

Plantar pododermatitis

405 The plantar surface of the foot pads of broilers, broiler breeders and turkeys may become severely ulcerated and caked with litter. This is seen most frequently when the litter condition is poor, particularly if flocks are scouring.

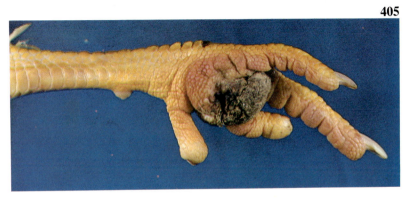

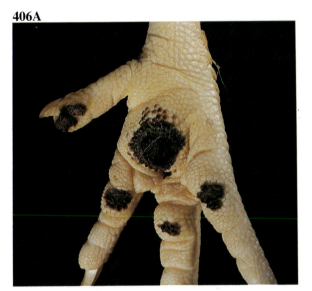

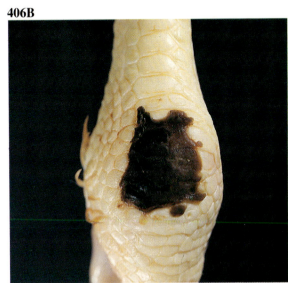

406 Lesions may also occur on the digits (**406A**) and – if there is sufficient contact with damp or caked litter – on the hock (**406B**) and the breast skin.

Ionophore toxicity

407 Severe myodegeneration of leg muscles may ensue, resulting in lameness, a reluctance to walk, and variable mortality. Muscles are selectively injured, with those of the thigh often containing lesions. Grossly, there is usually little significant change, but in severe cases the muscle fascia may be covered with a thin layer of gelatinous oedema. In this 14-week-old turkey the pallor and mottling of the thigh muscles were associated with myodegeneration, but severe histological lesions may exist in the absence of any distinct gross findings. However, in very acute cases, death may occur without there being any marked histological evidence of myodegeneration.

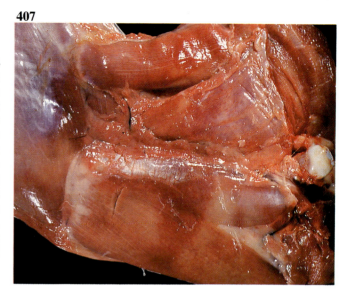

408 Myodegeneration affecting a thigh muscle in an 11-week-old turkey. Floccular changes are present in the necrotic sarcoplasm of the central fibre, and some phagocytosis is taking place. The lesion is not specific.

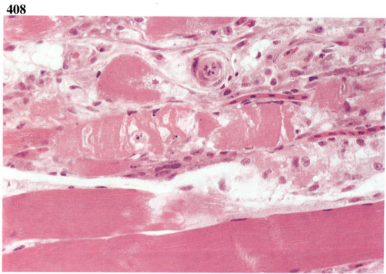

409 Punctate basophilic stippling caused by mineralisation is evident in the swollen degenerating fibre across the centre of the field. The lesion is uncommon and not specific. Turkey grower.

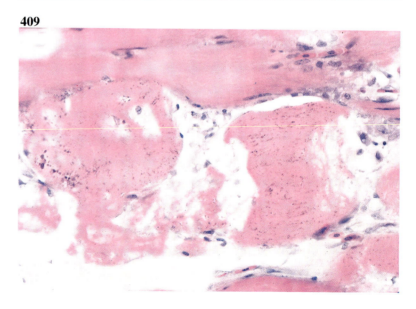

410 Punctate mineralisation in a degenerating muscle fibre of a turkey. Von Kossa.

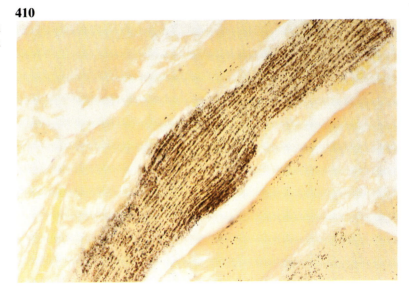

Tracheal and bronchial obstruction with asphyxiation

411 Obstructive lesions occur frequently at the syrinx or in the extrapulmonary primary bronchi. The syrinx (arrow) of this 14-day-old commercial layer chick is abnormally pale due to the accumulation of purulent debris in the lumen. The flock had been spray-vaccinated with a live respiratory virus vaccine at 8 days of age. In this instance the spray droplet size was probably too small. Obstructive lesions of this type may be seen in several respiratory infections (*see also* **131**, **135**).

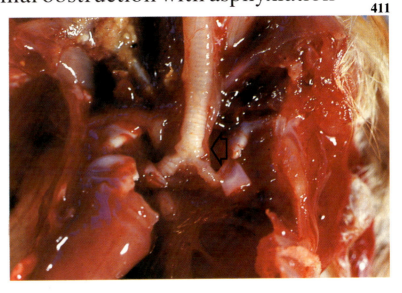

412 Plugs of exudate protruding from the severed ends of extrapulmonary primary bronchi in the same case as illustrated in **411**.

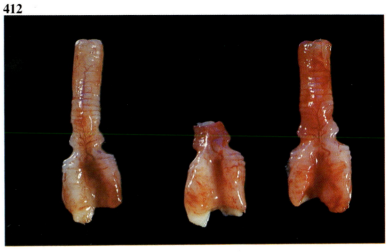

413 An extruded bronchial plug from a specimen shown in **412**. As a result of asphyxiation, the lungs of the chick in **411** were congested, which drew attention to their respiratory tracts.

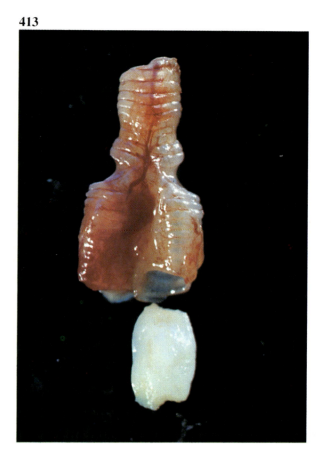

Swollen head syndrome

414 In Britain this syndrome has been associated in broiler breeders and broilers with exposure to the turkey rhinotracheitis agent (*see* **153**). Head swelling is produced by a cellulitis, from which *Escherichia coli* can frequently be isolated. The supra-orbital skin has been reflected in this specimen to expose the purulent subcutaneous reaction.

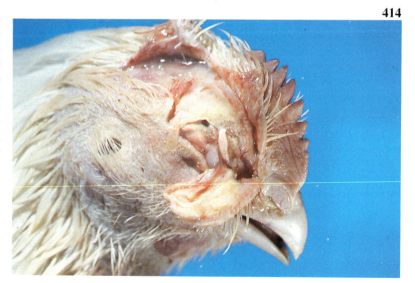

415 In birds exhibiting nervous signs there is usually an extensive purulent inflammation in the spongy bone of the neurocranium. A cross-section of this fixed skull has been taken through the cerebellum. The affected areas (arrows) are paler than the surrounding tissue.

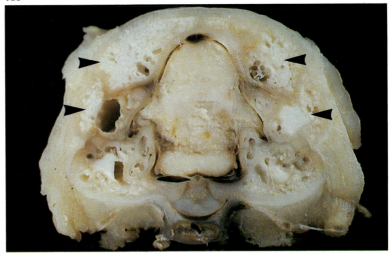

416 In this low-power view of the cranial spongy bone, the air spaces are full of purulent exudate. The deeper-staining exudate on the right has been established for longer than the inflammatory oedema on the left (arrow). Small clumps of bacteria are often seen in these lesions. Nervous signs are caused by labyrinthitis or by extension of the lesions to the meninges. Differential diagnosis should include consideration of the cranial form of fowl cholera (*see* **18**).

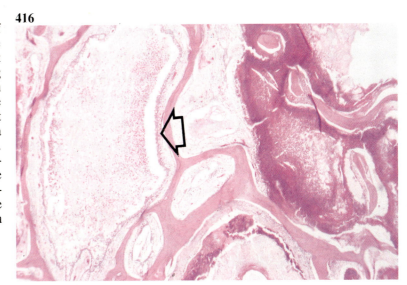

Gizzard erosion and ulceration

417 Thick and roughened gizzard lining in a commercial layer replacement pullet. Erosions and ulcers are present. This type of lesion is more common in broilers and is occasionally seen as an outbreak.

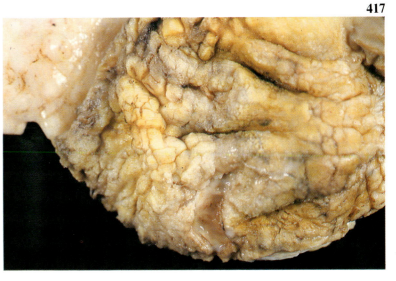

418 The surface of this gizzard from a 6-week-old broiler is covered with thick blood-stained material, haemorrhage having occurred from a large central ulcer. Changed blood arising from this source may be found in the crop and the proventriculus, also in the intestine.

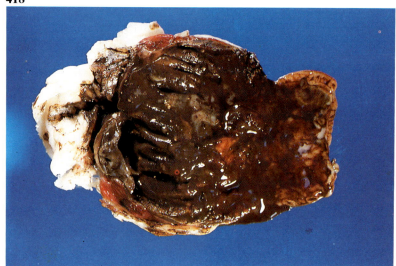

419 Sections usually exhibit an irregularly thickened and loosened lining, which often stains poorly. Note here that some of the gizzard glands have been lost and that inflammation extends into the muscularis. Frequently, the disordered gizzard lining contains many desquamated glandular cells and degenerating granulocytes.

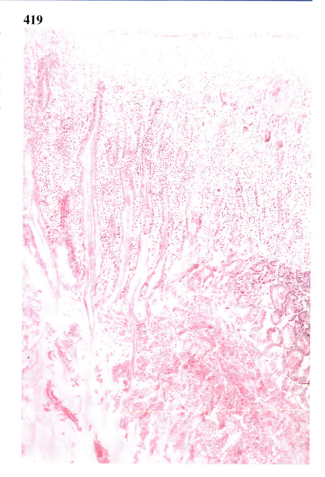

Aortic rupture in turkeys

420 The abdominal aorta is most often affected. A large blood clot is present in the abdominal cavity of this 17-week-old male bird.

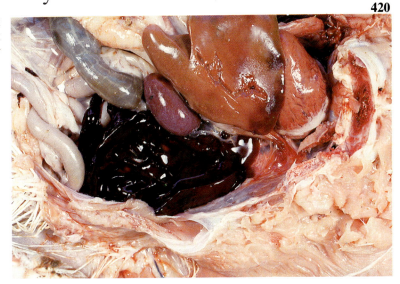

421 Cross-section of fixed tissue obtained from the specimen in Figure **420**, showing the ruptured arterial wall. Such lesions may be associated with atherosclerosis and aneurysm formation, although these changes were not observed histologically in this bird.

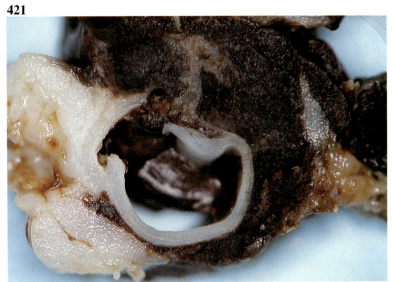

Corneal ulceration (keratoconjunctivitis)

422 Often referred to as 'ammonia blindness', lesions are most frequently seen in fowls being reared on deep litter. The ulcers, which may be unilateral or bilateral, are usually central and have irregular margins. This eye was fixed in Bouin's fluid before being photographed.

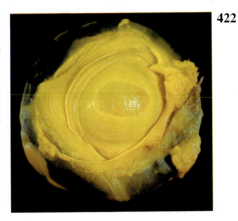

423 The ulcers are shallow and rarely breach Bowman's membrane (arrow). The epithelium tends to lift at the margin and one such tag is shown. Mild cellular infiltration of the cornea is often accompanied by a purulent conjunctivitis of varying severity.

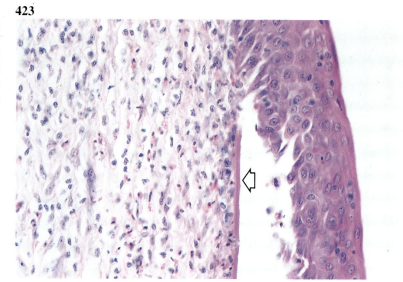

Persistent right oviduct

424 Cystic dilation of this structure (indicated by a blue pointer) is a common incidental post-mortem finding.

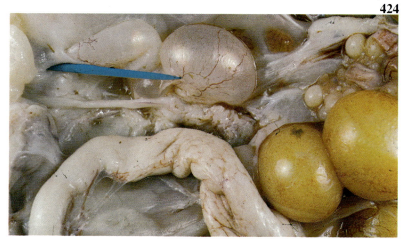

425 In some cases the cystic remnant may become very large and compress the abdominal viscera, with death possibly resulting. The abdomen of this layer is greatly distended by such a cyst.

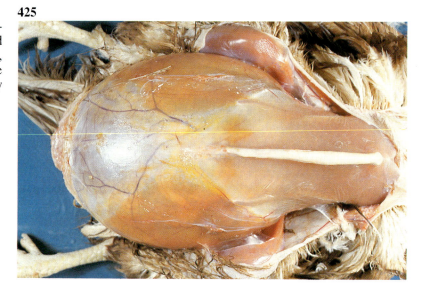

Internal layer

426 Three large soft-shelled eggs were found in the abdomen of this commercial layer, constriction of the magnum at one point having prevented their normal passage through the oviduct. Several more eggs are retained within the duct. Either soft- or hard-shelled eggs are occasionally found within the abdominal cavity of laying fowl that possess patent oviducts, and these may be adherent to the peritoneum.

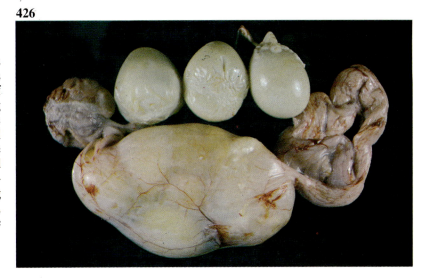

Prolapse of the oviduct

427 The lower part of the oviduct is protruding through the vent.

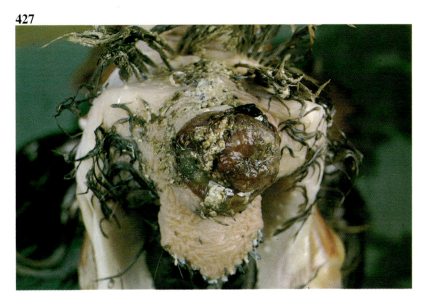

Cannibalism

428 In laying fowl the vent is most frequently attacked. At post-mortem examination most carcases are pale and have usually part or all of the intestines and reproductive tract missing.

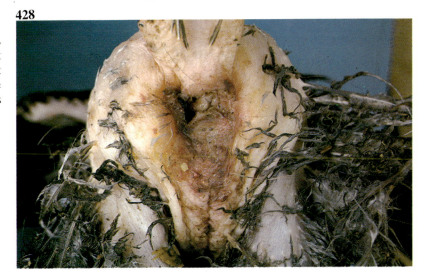

Poor thriving in chicks and poults

429 Failure to thrive as a result of adverse environmental conditions is a common cause of death at 5–7 days of age. The pectoral musculature is very thin in this chick.

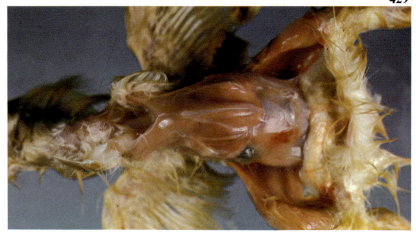

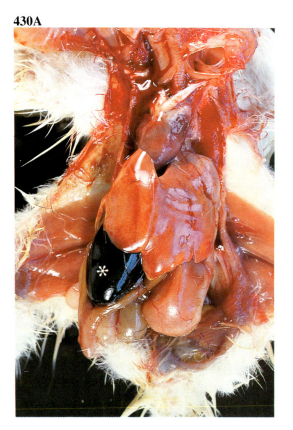

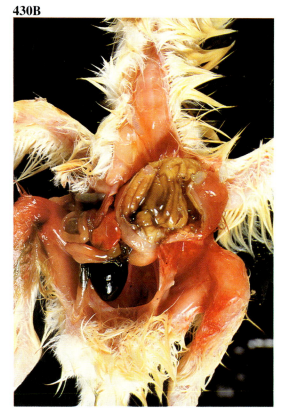

430 A distended gall bladder (asterisk) extends well beyond the posterior boundary of a pale liver in a turkey poult (**430A**). The empty gizzard has been opened (**430B**). The horny lining of the gizzard is often stained with bile. Yolk sac absorption is usually advanced.

431 Although the quantity of fat within the liver of birds under 1 week of age is normally high, hepatic sections from specimens that have not thrived reveal an excessive amount of lipid. Oil red O.

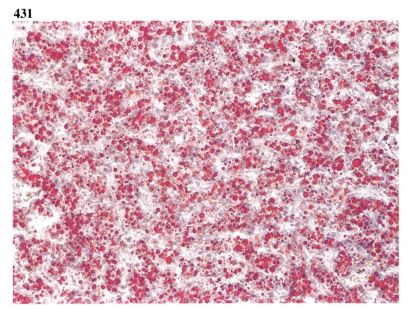

Pasted vent

432 The adhesion of a mass of excreta to the vent and nearby feathers can obstruct the subsequent passage of faeces and lead to death. A distended and impacted rectum can be seen in this 8-day-old chick. The kidneys of such birds are pale due to the retention of urates and interference with the outflow of urine. Vent pasting is usually associated with diarrhoea or a change in consistency of the faeces.

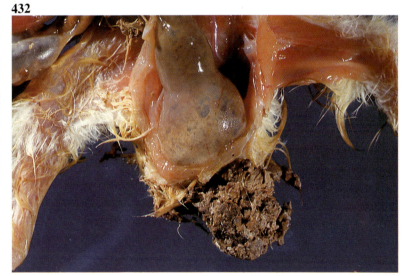

SELECTED READING

Calnek, B.W., Barnes, H.J., Beard, C.W., Reid, W.M. and Yoder, H.W. (Eds) (1990) *Diseases of Poultry*, 9th edition, Iowa State University Press.

Coutts, G.S. (1987) *Poultry Diseases under Modern Management*, 3rd edition, Nimrod.

Jordan, F.T.W. (Ed) (1990) *Poultry Diseases*, 3rd edition, Baillière Tindall.

Riddell, C. (1987) *Avian Histopathology*, American Association of Avian Pathologists, Inc.

Sainsbury, D.W. (1984) *Poultry Health and Management*, 2nd edition, Granada.

INDEX

References in this index are to figure numbers.